Guide to *Healthy* Fast-Food Eating

2nd Edition

Hope S. Warshaw, MMSc, RD, CDE, BC-ADM

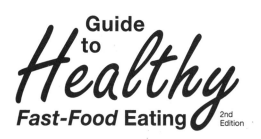

American Diabetes Association.
Cure • Care • Commitment®

Director, Book Publishing, Robert Anthony; *Managing Editor,* Abe Ogden; *Editor,* Rebekah Renshaw; *Production Manager,* Melissa Sprott; *Composition,* ADA; *Cover Design,* Vis-à-Vis Creative Concepts; *Printer,* United Graphics Inc.

Printed in the United States of America
1 3 5 7 9 10 8 6 4 2

ADA titles may be purchased for business or promotional use or for special sales. To purchase more than 50 copies of this book at a discount, or for custom editions of this book with your logo, contact the American Diabetes Association at the address below, at booksales@diabetes.org, or by calling 703-299-2046.

American Diabetes Association
1701 North Beauregard Street
Alexandria, Virginia 22311

Library of Congress Cataloging-in-Publication Data

Warshaw, Hope S., 1954-
  Guide to healthy fast food eating / Hope S. Warshaw. -- 2nd ed.
      p. cm.
  Includes bibliographical references and index.
  ISBN 978-1-58040-317-7 (alk. paper)
  1. Diabetes--Diet therapy. 2. Diabetics--Nutrition. 3. Fast food restaurants--United States. I. Title.
  RC662.W3152 2009
  616.4'620654--dc22

                    2009016828

To people with diabetes who, on a daily basis,
strive to control blood glucose to stay healthy
and prevent diabetes complications.
May the knowledge and information
you gain from this book help you
stay healthy and complication free.

–HSW

Contents

Preface

This compact and easy-to-carry *Guide to Healthy Fast-Food Eating* contains two main sections. In the first section, you'll learn how to eat healthier with diabetes (whether you are eating at home or away from home). You'll also gather skills and strategies on how to eat healthier in restaurants.

In section 2, you'll find a baker's dozen (13) of the top fast-food restaurant chains across the nation. This category of fast-food restaurants represents the most popular restaurants, with more than 100,000 locations worldwide. These are the restaurants that people frequent most often. They are also the category of restaurants for which the most nutrition information is now widely available.

In our fast-paced, convenience-focused world, it's likely that you'll continue to eat fast-food restaurant meals in your office, at home, or at the ball field. It's simply the way we are getting the job of eating done. With some skills, strategies, and nutrition facts in your hands, you can reach your goal to eat healthier; control your blood glucose, blood lipids, and blood pressure; and stay healthy for many years to come.

I encourage you to keep asking for nutrition information from any restaurant in which you dine and support legislation that is seeking to require restaurant chains to provide this information. If enough of us keep asking, eventually they'll give us the facts.

In health,

Hope S. Warshaw, MMSc, RD, CDE, BC-ADM

Acknowledgments

This book would have been impossible to create without the willingness of many large national and regional restaurant chains to be forthcoming with the nutrition numbers for their foods by making them available for the world to see on the Internet. To these restaurants, on behalf of the people with diabetes who will benefit from the information in the pages ahead, I am indebted. They set an example of consumer responsibility for the rest of the chain restaurant industry.

No book is completed by just the author alone. In this case, many manuscript pages and a large nutrient database became a book with many people's help. I am grateful to Paula Payne, RD, who assisted with the development of the nutrient database and other aspects of the book. Thanks also to all those at ADA who supported this effort: Rebekah Renshaw, Development Editor; Melissa Sprott, Production Manager; Abe Ogden, Managing Editor; and Rob Anthony, Director, Book Publishing.

And a last thanks goes to my professional colleagues who consistently lend their ears and ideas. They continue to be a source of inspiration and encouragement.

Section 1:
Healthy Restaurant Eating

Today's Diabetes Eating Goals

During the 1990s, diabetes eating goals underwent a minor revolution. In fact, the phrase "a diabetic diet" has become a misnomer. No such diet exists. No longer must you ax sugary foods and sweets from your list of acceptable foods. Now you can savor the taste of a few slices of pizza at your local pizza parlor or cruise to the drive-thru for a hamburger or grilled chicken sandwich when time is not on your side. The bottom line is that today's diabetes eating recommendations echo the healthy eating goals for everyone—whether the goals are from the government or respected health associations.

As a person with diabetes, you want to eat healthy to get to, and stay at, a healthy weight. You want to eat healthy to keep your blood glucose levels in the normal range as much as possible. Today, it's well known that eating and staying healthy with diabetes isn't just about blood glucose control. Recent research and recommendations suggest that you also get and keep your blood pressure and your blood lipids under control (check out the annually published *Standards of Medical Care for Diabetes* published each January within the *Clinical Practice Recommendations* found at www.diabetes.org).

Your diabetes eating and care plan should work around your needs and lifestyle and not vice versa. Your health care providers have many more medications and monitoring tools today to help you formulate a diabetes care plan that fits your lifestyle needs. The end goal, of course, is to keep you healthy and prevent or slow down long-term diabetes complications, such as eye, heart, and kidney problems.

Diabetes Eating Goals in a Nutshell

The latest American Diabetes Association (ADA) *Nutrition Recommendations and Interventions for Diabetes* put forth these key goals:

1. Achieve and maintain healthy **ABCs**

   A: Blood glucose levels in the normal range or as close to normal as is safely possible
   A1C: <7%
   Fasting and before-meals blood glucose:
   70–130 mg/dl
   2 hours after the start of a meal: <180 mg/dl

   B: Blood pressure levels in the normal range or as close to normal as is safely possible:
   At or under: 130/80 mmHg

   C: A [blood] lipid and lipoprotein profile [includes total cholesterol, LDL cholesterol, HDL cholesterol, and triglycerides] that reduces the risk for vascular disease [diseases of the blood vessels in the circulatory system]
   LDL: under 100 mg/dl
   HDL: above 40 mg/dl (men), above 50 mg/dl (women)
   Triglycerides: under 150 mg/dl

2. Prevent, or at least slow, the rate of development of the chronic complications of diabetes by modifying nutrient intake and lifestyle.

3. Address individual nutrition needs, taking into account personal and cultural preferences and willingness to change.

4. Maintain the pleasure of eating by only limiting food choices when indicated by scientific evidence.

Those are the key nutrition goals. But what foods should you eat to achieve them? Here are general pointers to focus on:

- Eat six or more servings of grains, beans, and starchy vegetables each day. Make at least three servings of whole grains.

- Strive for at least 2 1/2 cups of vegetables and 2 cups of fruit a day.

- Include two to three servings of fat-free or low-fat dairy foods each day—milk, yogurt, and cheese—within your calorie allotment. They provide calcium and other important nutrients. (Children, pregnant and breastfeeding women, and some adults have higher requirements for dairy foods.)

- Eat a moderate amount of meat and other protein foods. Two 3-oz servings each day are enough for most people. Not only does eating less meat help you eat less protein, it also makes it easier for you to eat less total fat, saturated fat, trans fat, and dietary cholesterol.

- Go light on fats and oils. Limit fats and oils high in saturated fat and trans fat, such as butter, cheese, solid shortenings, and partially hydrogenated fats, which contain trans fats. Trans fats find their way into restaurant food mainly in the frying oil (therefore fried foods). Limiting fried foods is a good way to limit trans fats, as well as many calories, when you eat in restaurants.

- Limit foods that contain cholesterol (such as red meats; seafood; poultry; whole-milk, full-fat cheeses; egg yolks; and organ meats).

- Enjoy small amounts of sugary foods and sweets once in a while. If you have some pounds to shed or your blood glucose or blood fats are not in a healthy range, eat sweets more sparingly. If you're on the slim side, you can splurge on sweets a bit more often if you want to as long as you can control your blood glucose adequately.

- Drink no more than one alcoholic drink a day if you are a woman and two drinks a day if you are a man. One drink is defined as 1 1/2 oz of hard liquor (a shot), 12 oz of beer, or 5 oz of wine.

To obtain detailed information about the amounts of foods you need based on your specific situation, consider consulting with a dietitian expert in diabetes care.

Everybody Sings the Same Song

ADA recommendations for healthy eating echo the recommendations from health organizations and government agencies. Whether it's the American Heart Association, the American Cancer Society, or the United States Department of Health and Human Services, they're all singing the same tune.

This means that as a person with diabetes, you don't need to stick out like a sore thumb because you strive to eat healthfully. There will be times that you'll feel like a fish swimming upstream because it's challenging to eat healthy restaurant meals and reasonable portions. It's not easy to eat healthfully. This is particularly true when it comes to restaurant foods—whether you are eating in or taking out.

How Much Should You Eat?

In order to make the long-term changes in your eating habits that will get and keep you healthy, you'll want to continue to eat at least some of the foods you have enjoyed for years, albeit in smaller quantities. The quantities of food you eat and when you eat need to match your lifestyle and schedule. Another critical element is to determine what foods and times for meals and snacks work best to help you keep your blood glucose, blood lipids, and blood pressure in control. Lastly, what's best for your diabetes is what allows you to feel good day to day and what helps prevent or slow down the development of diabetes problems.

No set number of calories or amount of foods or nutrients is right for everyone with diabetes. Your needs depend on many factors. A few of them are your height, your age, your current weight, and whether you want to lose weight or are at a healthy weight, whether you have a hard or easy time losing weight, your daily activity level, the type of physical activity you do, and more.

To develop an individualized eating plan and/or set healthy eating goals to make lifestyle changes, you may want to work with a registered dietitian (RD) with diabetes expertise, such as a certified diabetes educator (CDE). A dietitian can help support your efforts to change your eating habits over time.

Several books on the topic of food, nutrition, and meal planning published by the ADA give more in-depth information about how much and what you should eat (To order a book from ADA's extensive library of titles, visit *http://store.diabetes.org*).

Help Is Nearby

Whether you have just found out you have diabetes or you have been doing the diabetes balancing act for years, you can always learn more and benefit from a supportive diabetes educator. Get to know a diabetes educator. A diabetes educator will most likely be a nurse or dietitian but could be a pharmacist or exercise physiologist. Many diabetes educators have obtained the Certified Diabetes Educator (CDE) credential. A diabetes educator can help you tailor your diabetes management plan and offer tips for dealing with diabetes. The following resources are a good start to link you up with quality diabetes care:

- To find a Recognized Diabetes Education Program (a teaching program approved by the American Diabetes Association at which one or more diabetes educators work) near you, call 1-800-DIABETES (1-800-342-2383) or go straight to *http://www.diabetes.org/education/eduprogram.asp*.
- To find diabetes educators near you, call the American Association of Diabetes Educators (AADE) toll-free at 1-800-TEAMUP4 (1-800-832-6874) or go to *www.aadenet.org* and go to "Find an Educator."

It's now easier than ever for you to take advantage of the services of a diabetes educator or diabetes self-management education (DSME) as well as medical nutrition therapy (MNT) services from an RD under Part B Medicare services. Medicare has been covering DSME and MNT since the early 2000s for people with diabetes. Also, in nearly all states across the country, private insurers and managed care organizations that are regulated by the state must cover DSME and MNT. It's best to check with both the health care provider from whom you want to receive these services and your health care plan to determine the details on this coverage and ask if you need a referral.

Restaurant Pitfalls and Strategies for Self-Defense

Eating out healthfully is no easy task. It's downright challenging! You need willpower and perseverance. It's tough enough to eat healthfully in your own house, but even more challenges confront you when you are not able to control the portions or the condiments. You can't march into a restaurant's kitchen and hold the cook's hand while they ladle on more butter, slather on more mayonnaise, or shake more salt onto your once healthy foods.

Healthy restaurant eating is a challenge because of numerous pitfalls—from huge portions to the use of large quantities of fats, oils, sugar, and salt. Don't despair. You can learn to *choose* to eat healthfully in 99% of restaurants. To help make it easier on you, it's important to learn the pitfalls of restaurant eating. You'll find these discussed below. Next, you'll want to become well versed on healthy eating strategies. As you thumb though the tips and tactics in the pages ahead, you'll note that these strategies emerge repeatedly.

Pitfalls of Restaurant Eating

- **You think of restaurant ventures as special occasions.** Yes, once upon a time, people only ate in restaurants to celebrate a birthday, Mother's Day, or an anniversary. Not today. According to the latest statistics from the National Restaurant Association, the average American eats six meals away from home each week. And you may easily top that number. When you eat that many meals away from home, your waistline can quickly spread if you treat each meal as a special occasion. So, do you give up restaurant foods? There's no need to take that drastic step. Plus, depending on your schedule, cutting out eating out may not be possible for you. Today, restaurant meals for most people are just part of your fast-paced life and no longer just special occasions.

- **You're not the cook.** Your methods to control both portions and how your food is prepared are to ask questions about the food on the menu, to make special requests to get an item delivered the way you want it, and to practice portion control when you order and when you eat. Yes, assertiveness will be required!

- **Fats are here, there, and everywhere.** Remember, fat makes food taste good and stay moist. Restaurants love it. Fat is in high-fat ingredients, such as butter, sour cream, or cream; in high-fat foods, such as cheese, bacon, or potato chips; and in high-fat cooking methods, such as deep-fat frying, breading and frying, and sautéing. It's also at the table in the form of fried Chinese noodles, tortilla chips, or butter or oil for breads. You need to master the craft of being a fat sleuth. You'll get plenty of tips ahead.

- **Sodium can skyrocket.** Along with fat, salt makes food taste good. Salt or high-sodium preservatives are also used in many pre-prepared restaurant foods to keep them safe. Sodium can be particularly high in fast-food restaurants and others that use pre-packaged foods. It's nearly impossible for you to cut the sodium count of pre-packaged foods. The sodium can also be high in restaurants that prepare food from scratch, simply because they maximize taste by lathering the food in salt. Some ethnic foods, particularly Asian cuisines, can be high in sodium because of seasonings and sauces, like soy and teriyaki sauce. If you're watching your sodium intake, you will need to learn the ingredients and preparation methods that boost sodium and know where and how you can make reasonable special requests.

- **Portions are oversized.** Restaurants simply serve too much food. Unfortunately, we've evolved to a value = volume proposition in restaurants. Portions of food, particularly those produced and provided inexpensively, such as chips, fries, and drinks, are often enough for two. If there's one place to focus your attention and slowly change your behaviors, it's to develop and implement strategies that help you to not overeat. Hopefully you have a few willing dining partners in your midst.

- **Meat (protein) is front and center.** A primary focus of the American diner is summed up in the catchphrase "Where's the beef?" Whether it is fish, chicken, or beef, the "meat" or main source of protein often takes center stage, particularly in restaurant meals. For example, a portion of red meat in table service restaurants is often 8 oz or more cooked. (It's easier to order just-right portions of meats in fast-food restaurants by sticking with those small portions.) A chicken breast is often a whole chicken breast. A goal to eat healthier is to think about moving meat from front and center to the side where the portion takes up only one-quarter of your plate. Fill about half of the rest of your plate with vegetables and the other quarter with whole-grain starches. Yes, a goal to strive for, but not easy to do with restaurant meals!

Americans Eat Out: How Much and How Often?

According to the National Restaurant Association, in 1950 the average American spent only a quarter of his or her food dollar eating away from home. Today, an average American spends about half of every food dollar on food eaten away from home. Americans eat about one-third of their calories away from home, and eat six meals out of the house each week. Lunch is the meal eaten out most often, with dinner a close second. Breakfast is eaten out least often (keep in mind it is also the meal skipped most often, though it is known that eating breakfast has been shown to help people maintain weight losses.) Men eat out more than women. Fast-food restaurants, or walk up and order restaurants (as this book defines them)—from hamburger joints to pizza and sub shops—represent about a quarter of all restaurants. As for ethnic food, Americans' favorites are Mexican, Chinese, and Italian.

Let's face it, restaurant meals are just part of dealing with our fast-paced world. You might ask, "Is that a problem if I have diabetes?" The answer is no. Millions of people with diabetes eat restaurant meals. The challenge to people with diabetes is making healthy choices and eating reasonable portions…at least most of the time. And remember, whether you eat in the restaurant or take food out to the soccer field, your office, or the kitchen table, you face the same decisions. In fact, you have to make similar choices in today's supermarkets, because they have begun to look a bit like restaurants, with ready-to-eat parts of meals, complete meals, sandwiches, salads, and salad bars. One advantage to the supermarket is that the nutrition facts constantly stare you in the face. Not so in restaurants. At best, you have to have consulted the pages ahead and made decisions before you cross the threshold of the restaurant.

Ten Strategies to Eat Out Healthfully

1. **Develop a can-do attitude.** Too many people think in negative equations: Eating out equals pigging out; a restaurant meal is a special occasion; or eating out means blowing your "diet." These attitudes defeat your efforts to eat healthfully before you even start to try. Get ready to develop a can-do attitude about restaurant meals. Slowly begin to change how you order and the types of restaurants in which you choose to eat.

2. **Decide when to eat out—or not.** Take a look at how often you eat out. If your count verges on the excessive—at least once a day—then ask yourself why you eat out so frequently and how you can reduce your restaurant meals. If you reduce the restaurant meals you eat, you'll more easily eat healthier. Also, if you eat out more frequently, you need to keep splurges to a minimum. If you eat out only once a month, you might take a few more liberties—perhaps with an alcoholic drink or a dessert you split.

3. **Zero in on the site.** Seek out restaurants that offer at least a smattering of healthier options. If not, you'll set yourself up for failure. Believe it or not, there is an advantage to eating in chain restaurants.

You know the menu all too well. This can help you plan ahead, no matter which one of the chain's locations you pop into.

4. **Set your game plan in place prior to arrival.** On your way to the restaurant—whether it's a quick fast-food lunch or a leisurely weekend dinner—envision a healthy and enjoyable outcome. Plan your strategy, or at least what you might have if you aren't familiar with the restaurant. Don't become a victim of hasty choices or be swayed by the sights and smells that come your way.

5. **Become a fat sleuth.** Learn to focus on fats and the calories within. Fat is the densest form of calories, and it often gets lost in the sauce, on the salad, on the bread, or in the chips. Watch out for high-fat ingredients—butter, cream, and sour cream. Be alert for high-fat foods, such as cheese, avocado, or sausage. Steer clear of high-fat preparation methods like frying of any kind. Look out for high-fat dishes—Mexican chimichangas, broccoli with cheese sauce, or stuffed potato skins, for starters.

6. **Let your healthy eating goals or food plan be your guide.** Choose foods with your healthy eating goals or plan in mind. For example, if you're trying to eat more vegetables, focus on how you can accomplish this. Try to fulfill each food group with menu items or substitute foods to make your meal complete. For instance, replace a serving of milk or a fruit serving, which are often hard to get in restaurants, with another starch serving so that you will keep

your carbohydrate intake consistent—an important diabetes goal.

7. **Practice portion control from the start.** The best way not to eat too much is to order less. Order with your stomach in mind, not your eyes. You need to outsmart the menu to get the right amount of food for you. Because practicing portion control is central to healthy restaurant eating, you'll get plenty of tips and tricks in the pages ahead.

8. **Be creative with the menu.** You outsmart the menu by being creative. You also control portions by being creative. Remember, no sign at the entrance says, "All who enter must order an entree." Take advantage of appetizers, soups, and salads; split menu items, including the entree, with your dining partner; order one or two fewer dishes than the number of people at the table and eat family or Asian style; or mix and match two entrees to achieve nutritional balance. For example, in a steak house, one person orders the steak, baked potato, and salad bar and the other orders just the potato and salad bar, and then they split the steak. In an Italian restaurant, one person orders pasta with a tomato-based sauce and the other orders a chicken or veal dish with a vegetable.

9. **Get foods made to order.** Don't be afraid to ask for what you want, even in a fast-food restaurant. Restaurants today need your business and want you back. Make sure your requests are practical— leave an item such as potato chips off the plate; substitute mustard for mayonnaise on a sandwich;

make a sandwich on whole-grain bread rather than on a croissant; or serve the salad dressing on the side. Restaurants can abide by these requests; however, don't expect to have your special requests greeted with a smile at noon in a fast-food restaurant or when you try to remake a menu item. Be reasonable and pleasant.

10. **Know when enough is enough.** Many people grew up being members of the "clean-plate club." Now you need to reserve a membership in the "leave-a-few-bites-on-your-plate club." To keep from overeating, don't order too much, order creatively, and push your plate away when you meet your calorie needs. Remember, take-home containers are at-the-ready in most restaurants.

Restaurant Dilemmas and Diabetes

Many people who eat restaurant meals have concerns about their health and need to ask questions. So, as a person with diabetes, your questions and special requests are nothing out of the ordinary, especially today. However, as someone with diabetes, you deal with dilemmas beyond just the food. You also deal with your schedule for blood glucose–lowering medications and your blood glucose control. This section provides you with guidance to manage these added challenges.

Delayed Meals

Delayed meals can be a big challenge if you take a diabetes medication that can cause your blood glucose to get too low (see Table 1, p. 20). For example, if you are used to eating lunch between 12 and 12:30 p.m., how can you safely delay your meal until 1:00 or 1:30 p.m. when your friends or business associates want to meet? Or what should you do if you want to dine at 7:30 p.m. on a Saturday night, when your usual dinner time during the week is 6:00 p.m.?

A big and positive change in the management of diabetes today is that there are new oral blood glucose–lowering medications and new types of insulin and other injectable medications that better mesh with the realities of life in the 21st century. Several of these medications help you and your health care providers work out a medication

TABLE 1 Diabetes Medications and Hypoglycemia

Blood glucose–lowering medications that can cause hypoglycemia	Diabetes medications that do not cause hypoglycemia*
Sulfonylureas (this category of medication is used alone, in combination with other medications, or as a combination in one pill): Amaryl (glimepiride), Glucotrol and Glucotrol XL (glipizide), DiaBeta, Glynase, and Micronase (glyburide) *Meglitinides:* Prandin (repaglinide) *d-phenylalanine:* Starlix (nateglinide) *Insulin:* all types	*Metformin:* Glucophage, Glucophage XR, Riomet (liquid), Fortamet *Alpha-glucosidase inhibitors:* Precose, Glyset *Thiazolidinediones* (TZDs or glitazones): Avandia, Actos *Dipeptidyl peptidase-4 inhibitors* (DPP-4): Januvia (sitagliptin), Onglyza (saxagliptin) [at FDA for approval] *Incretin mimetic:* Byetta (exenatide), Victoza (liraglutide) [at FDA for approval] *Amylin analog:* Symlin (pramlintide) *This is generally true, unless these medications are used in addition to or in a combination pill that includes one of the medications that do cause hypoglycemia.

schedule that best controls your blood glucose, while allowing you the flexibility you need to live your life in the manner that best suits your needs. What's important in developing a medication plan is that you communicate your lifestyle and schedule to your health care providers. If they don't know your habits, then they are less able to help you develop a medication plan that suits you. Speak up! Don't wait for them to ask because they might not.

The biggest concern in delaying meals is if you have taken a diabetes medication that can cause your blood glucose to go too low (see Table 1, p. 20) if you don't eat on time. Prior to the availability of new blood glucose–lowering medications and newer insulins, this was more of a concern than it is today. However, it is certainly still a concern for you if your blood glucose can get too low. If you take one or more of the medications that can cause low blood glucose, you need to pay special attention to your meal times.

Keep in mind that several of the newer diabetes medications that can cause hypoglycemia are rapid-acting, such as the insulins lispro (Humalog), aspart (Novolog), and glulisine (Apidra), and the oral pills Prandin and Starlix. Their job is to quickly lower your blood glucose after you eat. If you take one of these medications along with other medications that are not likely to cause low blood glucose, you should take these rapid-acting medications before you start to eat rather than at your usual meal time.

If you take a pre-mixed combination of insulin, such as 70/30 or 75/25, or take insulin twice a day, such as a mixture of NPH and regular insulins, it becomes more important for you to eat on time to prevent low blood glucose. A disadvantage of these insulin regimens is that they do not allow much flexibility in meal times. If you regularly need more flexibility in your schedule, talk to your health care provider about your needs.

Practical Tips to Using Rapid-Acting Insulin with Restaurant Meals

Today, more people who take insulin are using one of several flexible insulin regimens, either a longer-acting insulin with a rapid-acting insulin in a pen for meal coverage or an insulin pump. These so-called flexible insulin regimens can make insulin dosing for restaurant meals easier.

Recent observations suggest that rapid-acting insulin doesn't lower blood glucose as quickly as practitioners first believed when it came on the market in 1996. Today, most experts agree that the maximum blood glucose–lowering effect of rapid-acting insulin occurs closer to two hours after an injection rather than 45–60 minutes. If this is true for you, the optimal time to take rapid-acting insulin is about 10 to 15 minutes before you eat, rather than with the first bite or 15 minutes after you start to eat.

Another big key to blood glucose control is to give yourself enough insulin to cover the rise of blood glucose from the food you eat. Like many people, you may find yourself in a reactive mode when it comes to dosing insulin. This means that you take your insulin in response to high blood glucose rather than taking enough insulin before a meal to cover the rise of blood glucose in the hours after you eat. This is usually between two and four hours, depending on what and how much you eat and several other factors. Experts agree that it's much harder to bring high blood glucose back down into the normal range than it is to control the rise of blood glucose with sufficient insulin taken before the meal.

Although taking rapid-acting insulin 10 to 15 minutes before a meal and carefully calculating your dose according to the carbohydrate you will eat are ideal for blood glucose control, you may not always be able to do so when you eat restaurant meals. These practical tips can help you keep your blood glucose in better control when you eat restaurant meals:

High blood glucose before a meal: Take some rapid-acting insulin 30 minutes before your meal to give the insulin time to lower your blood glucose. It might take longer than this to come down, but at least it will be on the downswing.

Low blood glucose before a meal: If your blood glucose is low before a meal (below about 70 mg/dl), wait to take your insulin. Give some of the carbohydrate from your meal about 15 minutes to raise your blood glucose before you take the insulin to cover your food.

Uncertain carbohydrate intake: If you don't know how much carbohydrate you will eat at a meal, consider splitting your rapid-acting insulin dose. Take enough insulin 15 minutes before the meal (if your blood glucose is in an OK range) to cover a minimum amount of carbohydrate that you know you will eat, say 30 to 45 grams. Then, as the meal goes on and you know how much more carbohydrate you will eat, take more insulin to cover this amount. This method is easiest if you are on an insulin pump or if you use an insulin pen and don't mind an extra injection.

Drawn-out meals: Pump users who plan to have a long, drawn-out restaurant meal or a meal that is higher in fat may want to consider using one of the optional bolus delivery tools on their insulin pump. Most insulin pumps allow you to deliver a bolus over time rather than all at once or to deliver some insulin immediately and some over the next few hours.

Learn from your experiences: Because of the large variation in individual responses to blood glucose from food and insulin, learn how to fine-tune your control by recording your experiences for future reference. Keep notes of your responses to various foods and activities in a notebook, computer file, or logbook. Chart the following: foods you eat and the amounts, the amount of insulin you take to cover the food, your blood glucose levels before and after you eat (2 hours, 4 hours, and 6 hours), and any lessons you learn to apply when you eat a similar meal the next time around. Although controlling blood glucose is difficult, a personal database can help you adjust to many different situations you encounter in everyday life.

Steps to Take If Low Blood Glucose Is Possible

If you will delay a meal and you take a longer-acting pill or insulin that can cause your blood glucose to get too low, take precautions to prevent this. Follow these steps.

Check your blood glucose at the usual time of your meal.

- If it is high (>150 mg/dl), you can wait a short time before you eat without concern. Check again if you feel your blood glucose is getting too low before your meal.
- If your blood glucose level is around your pre-meal goal (70–130 mg/dl) and you feel it will fall too low before you get to eat, eat some carbohydrate (start with 10 to 15 grams) to make sure your blood glucose doesn't go too low before your meal.
- If you delay your meal more than one hour and your blood glucose is around your pre-meal goal, you may need to eat more than 10 to 15 grams of carbohydrate to keep it from going too low before your meal.

It is always a smart idea to keep quick and easy carbohydrate foods in places like your desk, briefcase, purse, locker, or glove compartment. Also, it is good to carry a form of pure glucose, such as tablets, gel, or liquid. They help you treat impending low blood glucose before it gets too low and are the most desirable and effective form of treatment for low blood glucose. After all, you never know what will happen in restaurants.

Suggested foods that are easy to carry and contain carbohydrate are dried fruit, cans of juice, pretzels, milk, yogurt, gum drops, gummy bears, or snack crackers. Check the nutrition facts label on the food to determine the amount equivalent to 15 grams of carbohydrate.

If your blood glucose is lower than 70 mg/dl and you feel the symptoms of low blood glucose, you should use 15 to 20 grams of some source of carbohydrate to treat your hypoglycemia. Try to eat your meal soon after.

These suggestions offer you general rules of thumb. Check with your health care providers or diabetes educator to learn the best alternatives for you based on your diabetes medication plan. If your diabetes medication plan is not fitting with your lifestyle, recognize that there are alternatives.

Alcohol

There are numerous reasons not to drink alcohol. Alcohol is high in calories (unhealthy calories); it can cause low blood glucose if you take an oral diabetes medication or insulin that can cause low blood glucose; and it can lead to health problems with overuse, can slow your responses, and can be dangerous if you drink and drive. However, if your blood glucose and blood lipids are in good control and you drink sensibly, there is no reason you cannot enjoy some alcohol. A common time to drink alcohol is when you eat in a restaurant. Here's how to drink smartly with diabetes.

TIPS TO SIP BY

- Don't drink when your blood glucose is below 70 mg/dl or you have symptoms of hypoglycemia.
- Remember that alcohol can cause low blood glucose soon after you drink it (if your medicine is working hardest and/or you need to eat). It can continue to cause low blood glucose 8–12 hours after you drink it, especially if you drink in excess, take too much medicine, or don't eat enough.
- Don't drink on an empty stomach. Either munch on a carbohydrate source (popcorn or pretzels) as you drink or wait to drink until you get your meal.
- Keep in mind that alcohol contains a concentrated source of calories and virtually no nutrition. If you have few calories to spare because you are trying to shed pounds or keep pounds off, there won't be much room for alcohol.
- Alcohol can also make blood glucose too high. This is true for anyone with diabetes, no matter how they control it. High blood glucose can be caused by the calories from carbohydrate in the alcoholic beverage, such as wine or beer, or in a mixer, such as orange juice.
- Avoid mixers that add lots of carbohydrate and calories—tonic water, regular soda, syrups, juices, and liqueurs.
- Check your blood glucose to help you decide whether you should drink and when you need to eat something.

- Wear (preferably) or carry identification that states you have diabetes. Keep in mind that signs of hypoglycemia can be mistaken for symptoms of being drunk.
- Sip a drink to make it last.
- Have a noncaloric, nonalcoholic beverage by your side to quench your thirst during a meal.
- If you do not have to lose weight, just have an occasional drink and don't worry about the extra calories.
- Do not drive for several hours after you drink alcohol and when you do get ready to drive, check your blood glucose and make sure it's in a healthy range. Never drink and drive!

Sugars and Sweets

It is common to want a sweet dessert to end a restaurant meal. As you know by now, you can fit sweets into your diabetes eating plan as long as you substitute them for other foods or compensate for their extra carbohydrate, fat, and calories with your blood glucose–lowering medicines to keep your blood glucose close to normal. To set healthy goals with sweets, you also need to consider your weight and blood fats. Work with a dietitian to figure out how to fit sweets into your healthy eating plan. In the meantime, here are a few pointers.

HINTS TO SATISFY YOUR SWEET TOOTH

- Prioritize your personal diabetes goals. Which is most important for you: blood glucose control, weight loss, or lower blood fats? Your priorities dictate how you strike a balance with sugars and sweets.
- Choose a few favorite desserts. Decide how often to eat them and how to fit them into your eating plan.

- Perhaps it is best for you to limit desserts to when you eat in restaurants. That way you keep sweets out of your home.
- Split a dessert in a restaurant or take half home if possible. Portions are generally too big.
- Take advantage of smaller portions available in restaurants or ice cream spots—kiddie, small, or regular are the words to look for.
- Use the nutrition information you find in this book and information you find in restaurants to learn about the calorie, carbohydrate, fat, saturated fat, and cholesterol content of desserts.
- When you eat a sweet, check your blood glucose about two hours later to see how it has been affected. Then check again at four or five hours to see if your blood glucose is back down to your pre-meal target. You might find, for instance, that because of the fat content, the same quantity of ice cream raises your blood glucose more slowly than does frozen yogurt, which contains less fat and more carbohydrate.
- Keep an eye on your A1C (your longer-range blood glucose measure) and your blood fat (lipid) levels to see whether eating more sweets leads to a worsening in these numbers.

These are basic guidelines and suggestions to deal with diabetes restaurant dilemmas. Each person with diabetes is different, so talk with your health care provider and diabetes educator to get information pertinent to the way you manage your diabetes.

Restaurants Can Help or Hinder Your Healthy Eating Efforts

The pendulum swings back and forth on how helpful restaurants are when it comes to efforts to provide healthier choices. During the 1980s and early 1990s, when the voices of people concerned about what they ate and about their health were loud, restaurants developed healthier options. Lower-calorie and lower-fat menu items were introduced. Restaurateurs willingly made lower-fat milk and reduced-calorie salad dressings available. Some restaurants even marked their menus with little hearts or other notations to indicate which menu items met specific health criteria.

The pendulum in restaurants then swung back in the late 1990s and early 2000s. McDonald's dropped the McLean hamburger and meal-sized salads. Belly-busting portions became commonplace again. Taco Bell's Border Lights line bombed because it was introduced toward the end of this round of the health craze. We were back in the era of triple-decker burgers, meal deals, and more all-you-can-eat buffets.

But then the pendulum swung again due to another round of interest in low-carb diets and, more important, a focus on childhood and adult obesity. Restaurant chains have responded in small ways. A few examples: McDonald's has stopped supersizing; several large hamburger chains are offering healthier side options including fruits and vegetables; Subway has taken on healthier eating in a big way, offering 6-inch subs and a handful of sandwiches with a minimal number of grams of fat; and, in many restaurants, it's easier to split and share items as well as get a range of items prepared your way.

Other interconnected movements are afoot in restaurant cuisine. One is the slow food movement, which promotes less processed and more made-from-scratch foods. Another is the push for restaurants to use more locally grown fruits and vegetables and meats raised and processed more humanely and without hormones. Additionally, organic items are finding their way onto menus.

Unfortunately, a majority of Americans still cast most health and nutrition cares to the wind when they set food in any restaurant. It's easy to see where that is leading us. Today, nearly two-thirds of American adults are overweight, nearly 24 million people have diabetes, and about 57 million more have pre-diabetes.

This "no cares" nutrition attitude makes it harder for people who are health conscious. But don't feel pessimistic. Lower-fat milk, reduced-calorie salad dressings, and a few healthier options are still widely available. There's also a greater ease in making special requests—ordering half portions and splitting items or meals down the middle with your dining partner. With skills and a bit of fortitude, you can eat healthfully at most restaurants. Granted, you still have to pick and choose among the menu offerings.

Chains That Give the Nutrition Lowdown

The restaurants included in this second edition provide complete nutrition information. The "walk up and order" type restaurants—pizza, chicken, Mexican and Chinese food, subs and sandwiches, donuts and bagels, and frozen desserts—provide the most complete nutrition information.

The types of restaurants that, for the most part, either do not have or do not provide nutrition information are chain sit-down restaurants. Several of these restaurants are all too happy to give you nutrition information about their healthier items; however, they either don't have, or are unwilling to disclose the nutrition information for the complete menu.

Why don't some restaurants provide nutrition information? There are a few reasons. First, it's expensive to obtain nutritional analyses on all menu items. Second, restaurants that do not provide information tend to change their menus frequently. As soon as they printed nutrition information, it would need to be revised. Third, they want you to stay blindfolded to the nutrition lowdown on their foods. An important point here is that you—a person with diabetes concerned about your health—need to keep asking for nutrition information at restaurants that don't give it.

How to Get the Latest Nutrition Lowdown

This book has just 13 restaurants. There are more fast-food and sit-down chain restaurants that provide nutrition information. Here are a few hints on how to get the nutrition information for these restaurants.

■ If you have access to the Internet, use it. Usually the nutrition information is tucked into the menu information.

- If you don't have Internet access, ask for nutrition information at the store location you frequent. You might get lucky and have a nutrition pamphlet put right into your hands. Make sure you check the date on the nutrition pamphlet to be sure it is current.
- If the restaurant does not have the information, ask where you can call or write for it. You might need to call or write the corporate headquarters and have them send you a pamphlet.
- If you have a question about the nutrition content or ingredients used in a few items, contact the company either through the Internet or by phone.

A Bit of Help from Your Government

The Nutrition Facts panel on most canned and packaged foods in the supermarket hardly seems new. It's now been around since about 1994. The Nutrition Labeling and Education Act (NLEA) changed the nutrition label, increased the number of foods with information, and required restaurants to comply with several aspects of this law. Restaurants must provide nutrition information to customers when nutrition and health claims are made on signs and placards. If any restaurant makes a health claim about a food, that it is "low-fat," for instance, the nutrition information has to comply with the meaning of that nutrition claim according to the NLEA. This helps you know that when you see the word "healthy" to describe a can of beans or a fast-food sandwich, it has the same meaning. Restaurants from small one-unit sandwich shops to McDonald's have to abide by these regulations. Table 2 (see page 34) provides terms you might see on restaurant menu items and their definitions.

The law permits restaurants to make:

- Specific claims about a menu item's nutritional content.
- One of the approved health claims about the relationship between a nutrient or food and a disease or health condition. The criteria to make the health claim must be met. (There are about 15 FDA-approved health claims. These are different than nutrition claims.)

If the restaurant makes a nutrition or health claim, it must provide you with the nutrition information to back it up. The claim can be substantiated by a nutrition database, nutrition information in the cookbook from which the recipe was made, or another source that provides nutrition information. Further, restaurants do not have to give you the information in the nutrition label format you are familiar with from the supermarket. They can provide it in any format they choose.

There is a move in a handful of cities and states to require chain restaurants with more than 20 outlets to provide some basic nutrition information, such as calories, saturated fat, trans fat, carbohydrate, and sodium at the point of purchase, such as right next to the price of the item on menus or menu boards (not just on their Internet sites, on posters, or in brochures available in the restaurants).

This is great news for people with diabetes because it's the key information you need to make wise choices. Legislation began to snowball in 2008 with New York City and Seattle putting legislation into action. In September 2008, California's governor signed a bill into law that requires restaurant chains to provide brochures with nutrition information in their

TABLE 2 **Meaning of Nutrition Claims on Menus, Signs, and Placards***

Nutrition Claim	Meaning
Cholesterol-Free	Less than 2 mg of cholesterol per serving and 2 g or less of saturated fat per serving
Low Cholesterol	20 mg or less of cholesterol per serving and 2 g or less of saturated fat per serving
Fat Free	Less than 0.5 g of fat per serving
Low Fat	3 g or less of fat per serving
Light/Lite	Cannot be used by restaurants as a nutrient content claim, but can be used to describe a menu item, such as "lighter fare" or "light size"
Sodium Free	Less than 5 mg of sodium per serving
Low Sodium	140 mg or less of sodium per serving
Sugar Free	Less than 0.5 g of sugar per serving
Low Sugar	May not be used as a nutrient claim
Healthy	The food item is low in fat, low in saturated fat, has limited amounts of cholesterol and sodium, and provides significant amounts of one or more key nutrients—vitamins A and C, iron, calcium, protein, or fiber.
Heart Healthy (These claims will indicate that a diet low in saturated fat and cholesterol may reduce the risk of heart disease.)	The item is low in fat, saturated fat, and cholesterol, and provides significant amounts (not added) of one or more key nutrients—vitamins A and C, iron, calcium, protein, or fiber. OR The item is low in fat, saturated fat, and cholesterol, and provides significant amounts of one or more key nutrients—vitamins A and C, iron, calcium, protein—and is a significant source of soluble fiber.

*The definitions of these claims are the same as those used for food labels in the supermarket. Learn more about nutrient claims and health claims at the U.S. Food and Drug Association website (www.fda.gov).

restaurants (this will start in July 2009 and take full effect in 2011). Federal, state, and city legislators in other areas are forging ahead to put this legislation into effect across the nation. Two bill have already been introduced in both the Senate and the House to enforce a national nutrition labeling policy in chain restaurants. Check out what's going on federally by searching the Internet for "restaurant nutrition labeling laws." Consider weighing in with your support of the legislation to your federal representatives.

Tips to Eat Healthier, from Breakfast to Burgers, Pizza, and More

Healthy Tips for Breakfast and Snack Restaurants

- Choose coffee without cream, whole milk, or sugar. They add fat and empty calories. Use lower or fat-free milk and sweeten with a sugar substitute. Today you often have three choices—Splenda, Equal, and Sweet 'N Low.
- Try half of a soft-baked pretzel as an accompaniment to a salad or as a snack.
- Opt for one of the light bagel spreads, but keep in mind that they are hardly calorie or fat free. Spread them thinly.
- Cake donuts have slightly less fat than yeast donuts.
- Consider a half of a bagel, muffin, scone, or sweet bread. For many people, that's enough carbohydrate and calories. If a whole-grain variety is available, grab it.
- Eat breakfast. Skipping breakfast just keeps your engine in low gear and may help you rationalize overeating at meals during the rest of the day. Plus, if you take diabetes medications that can cause low blood glucose, skipping breakfast is not a smart move.

- In breakfast sandwiches, choose ham or cheese and pass on bacon or sausage. Have these fillings on a bagel or English muffin rather than the high-fat biscuit or croissant.
- Read the fine print when you see the words "low-fat," "fat-free," or "sugar-free." They don't mean that there are no calories or no carbohydrate. In fact, some of these foods can contain more carbohydrate and/or more calories than the regular food.
- If jam or jelly is an option, take it. Jams and jellies have no fat. Spread them thinly all the same.
- The fancy coffees and teas—both hot and iced, from mochas to frappuccinos to chais—are not just the coffee and tea. The whole milk, half and half, or whipped cream are just added calories and fat. The sugar from syrups adds calories and carbohydrate with no nutrition. These drinks can contain upwards of 300 calories for even the small size. You've got better ways to spend your calories.

HOW TO GET IT YOUR WAY

- Order bagel spreads on the side so that you can control how much is spread.
- Order butter or margarine on the side.
- Opt for fat-free milk in specialty coffees.
- Order a sandwich on a bagel or roll, not on a high-fat croissant.

Healthy Tips for Burger Chains

- Zero in on the words regular, junior, small, or single. These mean small portions.

- Try lower-calorie ketchup, mustard, or barbecue sauce as an option to higher-fat mayonnaise or special sauce.
- Limit the high-fat toppers—cheese, bacon, and special sauce.
- Look for healthier items—entrée and side salad, baked potatoes, healthy soups, cut fruit, and 100% juice.
- Walk in rather than drive through. If you eat and drive, you hardly realize food has passed your lips.
- Order less food to start. Remember, you can go back and get more in a flash.
- Want fries? Go ahead, but split a small or medium order.

GET IT YOUR WAY

- Avoid the busy times. This way you'll get your food your way with a smile on the order taker's face.
- Be ready to wait. Fast-food restaurants are not set up for special requests.
- Ask for simple changes: leave off the special sauce or mayonnaise; hold the pickles, bacon, or cheese; or hold the salt on the French fries.

Healthy Tips for Chicken Chains

- You are better off going skinless. If the chicken is served with skin, take the skin off and save some fat grams. You'll also lighten up on cholesterol and saturated fat.
- If there's enough for two meals, ask for a take-out container and split the meal into two before you dig in.

- To keep fat grams and calories down, go with the quarter white meat. Wings and thighs have the most fat.
- Order à la carte to pick and choose between the healthier items—piece of white meat chicken, corn, beans, etc.—skip the biscuit, hushpuppies, and other high-fat side items.
- If you are going to eat the meal at home, a better buy (price and healthwise) is a whole chicken and several sides. That way you—rather than the server—can decide on your portions.
- Split a quarter of a chicken meal and add an extra side or two. This keeps the protein portion where it should be, about 2–3 ounces.

GET IT YOUR WAY

- Ask to have the skin removed if you can't trust yourself to do it.
- Ask the server to take the wing off the breast.
- Ask for the gravy, butter, or salad dressing on the side.

Healthy Tips for Pizza Chains

- If you need to count calories carefully, stick with the thin crust and load up on the veggies.
- If your favorite chain does not publish nutrition information, check the nutrition information for similar items from two other pizza chains. This will give you ballpark figures to base your choice on.
- If your dining partner wants not-so-healthy pizza toppings, order healthier toppings on one half and let your partner handle the other.

- If you count grams of carbohydrate, make sure the slices you eat are average. If they are bigger or smaller, change your carbohydrate estimate and insulin dose (if you take insulin) based on your best guess for the size slices you eat.
- Order just enough for everyone at the table, to avoid that just-one-more-piece syndrome.
- If you know a few extra pieces will be left over, package them up before you take your first bite.
- Try an appetizer side portion of pasta, split an order with your dining partner, or stash a portion in a take-home container before you lift your fork to your mouth.
- Along with pizza or pasta, crunch on a healthy garden salad to fill you up and not out.
- The red pepper flakes you'll probably find sitting right on your table add zip to your pizza, pasta, or salad without adding calories.

HEALTHY PIZZA TOPPINGS

part-skim cheese	onions
sliced tomatoes	broccoli
chicken	Canadian bacon
green peppers	mushrooms
spinach	pineapple
ham	

NOT-SO-HEALTHY PIZZA TOPPINGS

extra cheese	several types of cheese
pepperoni	sausage
anchovies	bacon

GET IT YOUR WAY

- Ask your pizza maker to go light on the cheese and heavy on the veggies.
- Request a half-order of pasta if you don't have someone to split it with.
- Remember to order your salad dressing on the side.

Healthy Tips for Sandwich and Sub Shops

- Opt for the smaller size sandwiches when possible—6-inch sub, small, or regular size sandwich.
- To keep your sodium meter on low, go light on or hold the pickles and olives.
- To keep the fat level down, skip the oil and mayonnaise. Opt for vinegar and mustard. You get lots of flavor with next to no fat.
- Choose to have your sandwich made on whole-grain bread if it's available.
- Complement a sub or sandwich with a healthier side than a fried snack food (potato chips, tortilla chips, and the like). For some crunch, try a side salad, popcorn, baked chips, or pretzels.
- Ask to have large subs cut into two. Pack up half for another day.
- In sandwich shops, order a cup of broth-based vegetable or bean soup or a side garden salad. They'll fill you up and not out.
- A Greek salad and piece of pita bread make a moderate-carbohydrate and light-on-protein meal. Ask for dressing on the side.
- Pack a piece of fruit from home to bring to the sub or sandwich shop or enjoy it later.

GET IT YOUR WAY

- Hold the mayonnaise and oil. Substitute mustard or vinegar.
- Ask the sub maker to go light on the meat and heavy on the lettuce, onions, tomatoes, and peppers.
- Hold the cheese.
- Ask for the salad dressing on the side.

Healthy Tips for Mexican Restaurants

- If the fried tortilla chips greet you when you sit down, hands off. Send them back or at least to the opposite side of the table.
- Order à la carte to have less food in front of you and to pick and choose among the healthier offerings.
- Use extra salsa and other hot sauces to add flavor with very few calories.
- Use salsa or hot sauce as a salad dressing.
- Don't feel you have to order an entree. Choose from appetizers and side dishes to control your portions.
- As a starter, try a cup of black bean soup or chili to fill you up and not out.
- Make a bowl of black bean soup or chili the main course with a salad on the side.
- Look for menu items that use soft tortillas rather than crispy fried ones. For example, choose a burrito or an enchilada rather than a taco or a chimichanga.
- Fajitas are great to split. There's always enough for two.
- Split a side dish—Mexican rice, refried beans, or black beans—to get more carbohydrate and fiber.
- Take advantage of light or nonfat sour cream if it's served.

GET IT YOUR WAY

- Hold the guacamole, cheese, and sour cream, or ask for them on the side.
- If a menu item is served with melted cheese, request a light helping.
- Substitute black beans for refried beans (if available).
- Ask for extra tomatoes and lettuce.
- Request extra salsa or other zesty, low-calorie topper.

Healthy Tips for Ice Cream Shops

- Choose among the healthier toppings—fresh fruit, granola, nuts, or raisins.
- Take advantage of the variety of portions—from kiddie to multiple scoops.
- Don't think kiddie size is just for kids. It's a great small size for calorie and carbohydrate counters too.
- Order one dessert and two spoons. Just a few bites often quiets your sweet tooth.

GET IT YOUR WAY

- Low-fat or fat-free frozen yogurt, light ice cream, or sorbet are great options.
- Kiddie and small size options are aplenty for healthful eating.

Put Your Best Guess Forward

- Have measuring equipment at home and use it. Have a set of measuring spoons and measuring cups, as well as a food scale. There's a gamut of food scales available, from the inexpensive under $10 type, to expensive food scales that utilize an internal database to provide their nutrient counts based on the weight of the food. For more information on the more expensive scales, visit www.diabetesnet.com. If you are unfamiliar with portions, weigh and measure foods at home regularly to familiarize yourself with the portions you should eat. Then on occasion, weigh and measure foods, especially the starches, fruits, and meats. Weighing and measuring foods at home regularly helps you keep portions in control and can help you estimate them in restaurants. Estimating with the precise portion size helps you estimate the nutrient content correctly.
- Use these "handy" hand guides to estimate portions:
  - Tip of the thumb (to first knuckle)—1 teaspoon
  - Whole thumb—1 tablespoon
  - Palm of your hand—3 ounces (this is the portion size of cooked meat that most people need at a meal). Other 3-ounce portion guides: the size of a deck of regular size playing cards or the size of a household bar of soap.
  - Tight fist—1/2 cup
  - Loose fist or open handful—1 cup

Note: These guidelines hold true for most women's hands, but some men's hands are much larger. Check the size of your hands out for yourself with real weighing and measuring equipment.

■ Use the scales in the produce aisle of the supermarket to educate yourself about the servings of food you may be served in a restaurant, such as white or sweet potatoes, an ear of corn, a banana, or a half grapefruit. Weigh individual pieces of these foods. Check out how many ounces a potato or an ear of corn is that you may be served in a restaurant. Note that you are weighing these foods raw, but their weight doesn't change that much if they are served cooked.

■ If there are no data for a particular restaurant you frequent, use the information available from other similar restaurants. If you want to get a feel for the nutrient content of a food like French fries, baked potato, stuffing, pizza, or bagels, look at the serving size and nutrition information for those foods in restaurants that are included. You might want to take a few examples and then do an average. For example: if you regularly eat at a local pizza shop rather than a national chain and they have no nutrition information, take the nutrition information from this book for two slices of medium-sized regular crust cheese pizza from three restaurants. Then do an average. You will come pretty close to the nutrition content of the two slices of cheese pizza you eat.

■ You can also use the nutrition information from the nutrition facts of foods in the supermarket to estimate what you might eat in a restaurant. You might find some similar foods in the frozen or packaged convenience foods area. Again, take a couple of examples and then average.

■ If you regularly eat particular ethnic foods for which you find no nutrition information, you might want to get a few cookbooks out of the library (or use your own) that contain recipes for the foods you enjoy. Use a nutrient database or book with nutrition information to determine the estimated nutrient content for each ingredient. Do this for a couple of similar recipes. Get an average to help you estimate the nutrient content of what you are eating in the restaurant. This might work well for ethnic foods such as Indian, Mexican, or Chinese.

Most people regularly eat just 50 to 100 foods, including restaurant foods. People tend to frequent the same restaurants and order similar items. For this reason, it makes sense to spend a few hours estimating the nutrient content of your favorite restaurant items for which nutrition information is not available. Once you have this figured out, put it in a notebook, develop a computer file that you print out and keep with you, or put it into a personal data device that you always have with you.

Keep in mind that most restaurants serve portions that are larger than most average-sized people need to eat. So, even if you choose healthy foods that combine to make a healthy meal, you will likely also need to limit the amount you eat. Portion control is clearly not an easy task. Learn some techniques by reading the "Strategies for Self-Defense" on pages 11–18.

A word to the wise: avoid all-you-can-eat restaurants and other settings that promote overeating, such as hotel breakfast buffets or salad or food bars. This is best if you don't have much willpower or it bothers you to think that the restaurant is making money on you because you will not walk out feeling like a stuffed turkey. However, if you feel these settings work well because they help you control portions, use them to your advantage.

If you frequently eat particular items in a large chain restaurant that isn't in this book, contact the restaurant. Several restaurants note that while they don't provide nutrition information for all their items they would provide information for several items.

Even when you have consulted the nutrition facts for your menu items, practice defensive counting. Recognize that the nutrition information provided by restaurants is obtained from several samples of the foods prepared according to corporate specifications or based on the various ingredients. For this reason, on any given day, the portions of foods and ingredients you are served may be slightly more or less. Even in the fast-food hamburger chains, the same burger can include more or less ketchup, tomatoes, mayonnaise, or other ingredients. So, before you dig in, reassess your counts and ask yourself if the nutrition numbers provided by the chain add up based on your nutrition knowledge. If not, revise your counts.

Resources for Nutrition Information of Foods

BOOKS

Guide To Healthy Restaurant Eating, by Hope Warshaw, MMSc, RD, CDE, BC-ADM. American Diabetes Association, 4th edition, 2009. This book provides the calorie, carbohydrate, fat, and protein counts, along with full menus, for America's most popular chain restaurants. It also provides sample healthy meals and the healthiest bets for each restaurant.

The Ultimate Calorie, Carbohydrate, and Fat Gram Counter, by Lea Ann Holzmeister, RD, CDE. Small Steps Press, 2006. This book provides the carbohydrate count, as well as other nutrition information, for thousands of foods including fruits; vegetables and other produce; meats, poultry, and seafood; desserts; many foods you know by their brand name; frozen entrees; and more.

The Doctor's Pocket Calorie, Fat, and Carb Counter, by Allan Borushek. Allan Borushek and Associates (revised annually). This book lists calorie, fat, and carbohydrate information for thousands of basic and brand-name foods. (See www.calorieking.com to order the book or to download food and restaurant databases.)

Calories and Carbohydrates, by Barbara Kraus. Signet, 16th edition, 2005. Carbohydrate and calorie counts for more than 8,500 items are included in this food dictionary. It covers brand name and basic foods of every variety.

The Corinne T. Netzer Carbohydrate and Fiber Counter, by Corinne T. Netzer. Dell, 2006. This book features carbohydrate counts for thousands of foods, including fresh and frozen produce, dairy products, breads, grains, pastas, sweets, fast foods, and more.

INTERNET

www.diabetes/org/myfoodadvisor.html. This nutrient database, introduced in mid-2008, is provided for your use at no charge by the American Diabetes Association. It contains about 5,000 commonly eaten foods and for most of them provides the key nutrients: calories, carbohydrate, saturated fat, sodium, and fiber, as well as for several other nutrients and the percent daily value for some vitamins and minerals. There are many ways to use this searchable database to learn more about the nutrient content of foods and improve your food choices, such as searching for healthier alternatives, compiling the nutrient counts for your favorite recipes, or searching through the ADA's recipe box.

www.ars.usda.gov/ba/bhnrc/ndl. This is the U.S. federal government's nutrient database. It contains extensive nutrition information for about 7,000 basic and commercial foods. It is searchable and downloadable.

www.calorieking.com

www.healthydiningfinder.com. This is a joint venture between the Healthy Dining organization and the National Restaurant Association.

www.myfooddiary.com

www.nutritiondata.com

www.dietfacts.com

How This Book Works For You

Close but Not Exact

You should be aware that the nutrition information from restaurants is close but not exact. Many restaurants state that their nutrition information is based on the specified ingredients and preparation. However, the same restaurant has locations all over the country, and different regions purchase their ingredients and foods from different food wholesalers. For example, a Wendy's in California might purchase lettuce, tomatoes, and hamburger buns from one food supplier, whereas a Wendy's in Connecticut will buy foods from another company. The same is true internationally. When international chains make varied nutrition information available for their restaurants, the information used in this book were the U.S. figures. The nutrition analysis of these items is close, but not identical; however, it is close enough to help you to make food decisions and manage your blood glucose.

Restaurant foods are also prepared by different people. Even in the same restaurant, on different days you might get more or less cheese on your pizza, more pickles or ketchup on your hamburger, or a slightly smaller or larger steak, even though you order the 6-oz filet. Wherever humans are involved, portions aren't exact. Consider these differences if one day you notice that

your blood glucose goes up more or less than you expect from a restaurant meal you've eaten again and
again.

Beverages and Condiments

There are two categories of items that are not listed
separately in the information provided for each restaurant. The first is beverages. Regularly sweetened drinks,
such as carbonated beverages (soda), lemonade, non-
carbonated fruit drinks, as well as noncaloric beverages, milk, and 100% juice and the like, are not listed
repetitively within the information for each restaurant. The nutrition information for the most commonly served regular and diet beverages are found in
Table 3 on page 54.

The second category of items not repeated for each
restaurant is common condiments, such as ketchup, mustard, mayonnaise, and honey. Find this nutrition information in Table 4 on page 56. Information for items such as
salad dressing, barbecue sauces, and other special sauces
are provided within the specific restaurant.

The Nutrition Numbers Ahead

The nutrition information for the top 13 fast-food restaurants are in the pages ahead in the following order.

- Calories
- Fat (in grams)
  - Percentage of calories from fat. Look at this in re-
    lation to grams of fat. Keep in mind that the per-
    centage of calories from fat might be high, but
    the grams of fat might be low, or vice versa.

- Saturated fat (in grams). Saturated fat is the type of fat that raises blood cholesterol levels. Try to keep your saturated fat intake to 7% or less of your total calories.
- Trans fat (in grams). Trans fat is a type of fat that is saturated and unhealthy for your heart and blood vessels. It is mainly found in processed foods, but is also present in foods of animal origin, such as dairy foods, meats, poultry, and seafood. You are encouraged to eat as little trans fat as possible. (Trans fat is a new addition for the 2nd edition.) Due to the attention on trans fats and the inclusion of it on packaged food's nutrition facts since 2006, restaurants have felt the pressure to include it.

■ Cholesterol (in milligrams)
■ Sodium (in milligrams)
■ Carbohydrate (in grams)
  - Dietary fiber (in grams). Dietary fiber is a subcomponent of carbohydrate. Most people don't eat enough dietary fiber (less than 15 grams a day). You are encouraged to eat 20–35 grams of dietary fiber each day.
■ Protein (in grams)
■ Food servings/exchanges. The terms "servings" and "exchanges" are considered the same in this book (this is not true when it comes to the nutrition facts on food labels). Servings/exchanges have been calculated using the booklet *Choose Your Foods: Exchange Lists for Diabetes,* published by the ADA and the American Dietetic Association in 2008. A "best-fit" approach was used to calculate servings or exchanges.

TABLE 3 Nutrition Information for Beverages

Beverage	Amount	Cal.	Fat (g)	Sat. Fat (g)	Chol. (mg)	Sod. (mg)	Carb. (g)	Pro. (g)	Choices/Exchanges
Beer (regular)	12 oz	150	0	0	0	11	13	1	1 alc. equiv. + 1 carb*
Beer (light)	12 oz	103	0	0	0	18	5	1	1 alc. equiv. + 1/2 carb*
Wine, white	6 oz	120	0	0	0	7	1	0	1 alcohol equivalent
Wine, red	6 oz	125	0	0	0	6	4	1	1 alcohol equivalent
Coffee, black (regular and decaffeinated)	12 oz	4	0	0	0	7	0	0	free
Tea (hot, nothing added)	12 oz	4	0	0	0	7	1	0	free
Cola (regular)	20 oz	227	0	0	0	25	59	0	3 carb
Cola (diet)	20 oz	12	0	0	0	47	2	1	free
Soda, non-cola (regular)	20 oz	246	0	0	0	55	63	0	3 carb
Soda, non-cola (diet)	20 oz	0	0	0	0	95	0	0	free
Iced Tea (unsweetened)	12 oz	4	0	0	0	6	1	0	free

Liquor (any type)	1 1/2 oz	96	0	0	0	0	0	0	1 alcohol equivalent
Lemonade (regular)	12 oz	148	0	0	0	15	39	0	3 carb
Lemonade (sugar-free)	12 oz	11	0	0	0	14	2	0	free
Milk (whole)	8 oz	146	8	5	24	98	11	8	1 whole milk
Milk (reduced-fat/2%)	8 oz	122	5	3	20	100	11	8	1 low-fat milk
✓ Milk (low-fat/1%)	8 oz	102	2	2	12	107	12	8	1 fat-free milk, 1/2 fat
✓ Milk (fat-free)	8 oz	83	0	0	5	103	12	8	1 fat-free milk
Milk, chocolate (low-fat)	8 oz	160	3	2	8	152	26	8	1 fat-free milk, 1 carb
✓ Apple juice	8 oz	175	0	0	0	11	43	0	3 fruit
✓ Orange juice	8 oz	164	0	0	0	4	38	3	2 1/2 fruit

Source for nutrition information: U.S. Department of Agriculture, National Nutrient Database, http://www.ars.usda.gov. Consider the nutrition information as an estimate and not specific to the actual product you eat. If possible, use specific information when it is available.

*According to the calculation provided in *Choose Your Foods: Exchange Lists for Diabetes*, American Diabetes Association and American Dietetic Association, 2008. Talk to your diabetes educator or health care provider about how to work alcoholic beverages into your meal plan.

✓Healthiest Bets

TABLE 4 Nutrition Information for Condiments

Condiment	Amount	Cal.	Fat (g)	Sat. Fat (g)	Chol. (mg)	Sod. (mg)	Carb. (g)	Pro. (g)	Choices/Exchanges
Bacon, thinly sliced	1 slice	43	3	1	9	185	0	3	1 fat
Butter, stick	1 t	34	4	2	10	27	0	0	1 fat
Cheese, American	1-oz slice	105	9	6	26	416	0	6	1 high-fat meat
Cheese, Swiss	1-oz slice	95	7	5	24	388	1	7	1 high-fat meat
Cheese, mozzarella	1 oz shredded	85	6	4	22	178	1	6	1 medium-fat meat
Cream Cheese (regular)	1 T	51	5	3	16	43	0	1	1 fat
Cream Cheese (light)	1 T	35	3	2	8	44	1	2	1/2 fat
Half & Half, regular	2 T	39	3	2	11	12	1	1	1/2 fat
Honey	1 t	21	0	0	0	0	6	0	1/2 carb
Honey Mustard	1 t	7	0	0	0	16	1	0	free

Ketchup	1 T	15	0	0	0	167	4	0	free
Margarine (regular stick)	1 t	31	4	1	0	30	0	0	1 fat
Margarine (regular tub)	1 t	33	4	1	0	31	0	0	1 fat
Mayonnaise (regular)	1 T	57	5	1	4	105	4	0	1 fat
Mayonnaise (light)	1 T	49	5	1	5	101	1	0	1 fat
Mustard (regular)	1 t	3	0	0	0	57	0	0	free
Non-Dairy Creamer	1/2 oz/1 T	30	2	2	0	0	3	0	free
Olive Oil	1 t	40	5	1	0	0	0	0	1 fat
Pancake Syrup (regular)	1 T	47	0	0	0	16	12	0	1 carb
Pancake Syrup (light)	1 T	25	0	0	0	27	7	0	1/2 carb
Relish, sweet pickle-type	1 T	20	0	0	0	122	5	0	free
Salsa, tomato-based	1 T	4	0	0	0	96	1	0	free
Sour Cream (regular)	1 T	26	3	2	5	6	1	0	1/2 fat

(Continued)

TABLE 4 Nutrition Information for Condiments (*Continued*)

Condiment	Amount	Cal.	Fat (g)	Sat. Fat (g)	Chol. (mg)	Sod. (mg)	Carb. (g)	Pro. (g)	Choices/Exchanges
Sour Cream (light)	1 T	22	2	1	6	6	1	0	1/2 fat
Soy Sauce	1 t	2	0	0	0	340	1	0	free
Sugar	1 t	16	0	0	0	0	4	0	free
Teriyaki Sauce	1 t	5	0	0	0	228	1	0	free
Vegetable Oil	1 t	40	5	0	0	0	0	0	free
Vinegar (all types)	1 t	1	0	0	0	0	0	0	free

Source for nutrition information: U.S. Department of Agriculture, National Nutrient Database, http://www.ars.usda.gov. Consider the nutrition information as an estimate and not specific to the actual product you eat. If possible, use specific information when it is available.

There is not one right way to fit restaurant foods into your eating plan. Figuring out what food group the grams of carbohydrate come from is the biggest challenge to figuring servings or exchanges. This is how it was approached: When it appears that the grams of carbohydrate come from a starch—be it potato, bread, or starchy vegetable—the servings or exchanges are called starches. If the carbohydrate comes from vegetable, fruit, or milk, the servings or exchanges are designated as such.

A food group in *Choose Your Foods: Exchange Lists for Diabetes* is Sweets, Desserts, and Other Carbohydrate. This group contains sweets, frozen desserts, spaghetti sauce, jam, and maple syrup, to name a few. The calories and carbohydrate in many of these foods come from simple sugars. Therefore, in calculating the servings or exchanges for this book, we've called foods that fit into the "other carbohydrate" group "carb." Exchanges for fast-food shakes and frozen and regular desserts, for example, are calculated as carbs.

When it comes to meat dishes, the servings or exchanges were calculated based on the group that the meat fits into regardless of how it's prepared. For example, fish fillet sandwiches and chicken fingers are considered to fall into the lean meat group even though they have a lot of fat by the time they are served. On the other hand, sausage in any form is classified as a high-fat meat because that's the food group sausage fits into.

It is worth noting that several restaurants that provide nutrition information also provide exchanges. These were not used in this book. We calculated exchanges/servings based on ADA methodology. We have often found inconsistencies between the restaurant's exchange calculations and the ones obtained using ADA guidelines.

Putting It All Together

Perhaps one of the hardest parts of meal planning is figuring out how to put together healthy, well-balanced meals. This is a particular challenge in restaurants. To show you how to design healthier restaurant meals, we've put together two sample meals for most of the restaurants. In doing this, we've tried to show you variety and how you can mix and match foods to achieve your nutrition goals. We applied the following criteria to put together the meals. Please note that the criteria might be less strict than what you would consider for a healthy meal at home. That's because restaurant meals tend to be higher in calories, fat, and sodium.

In some restaurants, putting together healthier meals is easier, while in others it was virtually impossible to meet these criteria, especially for fat and sodium. Consider what the nutrition profile of meals in these restaurants would be if you weren't choosing with care. Also, keep in mind that you can make special requests to have higher fat or sodium ingredients left out, so that the items you eat are healthier.

An effort was made to minimize the amount of saturated and trans fat in all meals. This can be a challenge in restaurant meals. If you eat a restaurant meal that is high in fat and its components, balance this out with healthier meals other times of the day.

THE LIGHT 'N' LEAN CHOICE

- 400–700 calories (based on about 1,200–1,600 calories per day)
- 30–40% of calories from fat

- 100–200 milligrams of cholesterol (total per day should be 300 milligrams or less)
- 1,000–1,800 milligrams of sodium (total per day should be no more than 2,300 milligrams)

THE HEALTHY 'N' HEARTY CHOICE

- 600–1,000 calories (based on about 1,800–2,400 calories per day)
- 30–40% of calories from fat
- 100–200 milligrams of cholesterol (total per day should be 300 milligrams or less)
- 1,000–1,800 milligrams of sodium (total per day should be no more than 2,300 milligrams)

Healthiest Bets

With nutrition information in hand, we've made it easy for you to zero in on healthier restaurant offerings. We've marked these "Healthiest Bets" with a ✓. Remember, foods that are not marked as Healthiest Bets are not necessarily foods you should never eat. Healthiest Bets just steer you toward healthier choices.

When you're putting together healthy meals, don't look at only the Healthiest Bets. You can feel free to mix and match healthier and less healthy foods to make up overall healthy meals. Also keep in mind that if you split or share some less healthy bets, such as shakes, desserts, or fried items, they then fit into Healthiest Bets. That's why you'll see some Healthiest Bets and some less healthy items mixed and matched in the two sample meals for most restaurants. What's most important is that you eat a healthy balance of foods and meals over the course of the day and from week to week. So if you want a juicy hamburger and French fries for lunch one day a month, go ahead and enjoy.

The Healthiest Bets were chosen on the basis of the following criteria:

- Breakfast entrees: Less than 400 calories per serving, 45 grams of carbohydrate, less than 15 grams of fat (3 fat exchanges [about 30% fat]), and 1,000 milligrams of sodium.
- Lunch or dinner entrees, including entree salads: Less than 600–750 calories, 60 grams of carbohydrate, less than 20 grams of fat (4 fat exchanges [about 30% fat]), and 1,000 milligrams of sodium.
- Pizza, sandwiches (including breakfast sandwiches), hamburgers, etc.: Less than 500 calories per reasonable serving (for example, 2 slices of pizza), 60 grams of carbohydrate, 20 grams of fat (4 fat exchanges [about 30% fat]), and 1,000 milligrams of sodium.
- Side items: For items such as fruit, vegetables (raw and cooked), grains, legumes, starches, and meats, no more than 20 grams of carbohydrate, 5 grams of fat (1 fat exchange). For fried items, such as French fries, hash browns, chicken pieces, fried chicken, onion rings, and potato chips, less than 10 grams of fat (2 fat exchanges); less than 500 milligrams of sodium per serving.
- Soups: Less than 30 grams of carbohydrate, 10 grams of fat (2 fat exchanges), and 1,000 milligrams of sodium per serving.
- Salad dressings, cream cheeses, spreads, and condiments: Less than 50 calories, 10 grams of carbohydrate, 5 grams of fat (1 fat exchange), and 250 milligrams of sodium per tablespoon.

- Breads (such as rolls, biscuits, bagels, bread, croissants, scones, donuts, muffins, pretzels, and scones): Less than 400 calories, 45 grams of carbohydrate, 10 grams of fat (2 fat exchanges), and 800 milligrams of sodium per serving.
- Frozen desserts: Less than 300 calories, 30 grams of carbohydrate, and 10 grams of fat (2 fat exchanges) per serving.
- Beverages (such as milk, juice, milk shakes, and special coffees): Less than 300 calories, 30 grams of carbohydrate, and 5 grams of fat (1 fat exchange). Less than 400 milligrams of sodium. (Coffee and diet beverages, though minimal in calories, were not checked as Healthiest Bets.)

Bon appetit!

Section 2:
Fast-Food Restaurants

.

Arby's
(www.arbys.com)

Light 'n Lean Choice

Jr. Roast Beef Sandwich
Curly Fries *(1/2 small)*

Calories......................441	Cholesterol (mg).........29
Fat (g) 20	Sodium (mg)..........1,136
% calories from fat..41	Carbohydrate (g).........54
Saturated fat (g) 6	Fiber (g).....................4
Trans fat (g) 0	Protein (g) 18

Exchanges: 3 1/2 starch, 1 1/2 medium-fat meat, 2 1/2 fat

Healthy 'n Hearty Choice

Martha's Vineyard Salad with
Raspberry Vinaigrette *(1/2 packet, 2 T)*
Ham and Swiss Melt Sandwich

Calories......................638	Cholesterol (mg) 86
Fat (g) 21	Sodium (mg)..........1,845
% calories from fat..30	Carbohydrate (g).........69
Saturated fat (g) 7	Fiber (g).....................5
Trans fat (g) 0	Protein (g) 39

Exchanges: 3 starch, 1/2 carb, 3 veg, 4 1/2 lean meat, 1 1/2 fat

Arby's

	Amount	Cal.	Fat (g)	% Cal. Fat	Sat. Fat (g)	Trans Fat (g)	Chol. (mg)	Sod. (mg)	Carb. (g)	Fiber (g)	Pro. (g)	Choices/Exchanges
ARBY'S CHICKEN												
Chicken Cordon Bleu Sandwich - Crispy	1	590	26	4	5	0	76	1987	48	2	38	3 starch, 4 lean meat, 3 fat
Chicken Cordon Bleu Sandwich - Grilled	1	476	19	4	4	0	85	1725	37	1	43	2 1/2 starch, 5 lean meat, 1/2 fat
Chicken Fillet Sandwich - Crispy	1	510	24	4	4	0	52	1265	49	3	27	3 1/2 starch, 2 lean meat, 3 1/2 fat
✓Chicken Fillet Sandwich - Grilled	1	395	17	4	3	0	60	1002	38	2	32	2 1/2 starch, 3 lean meat, 1 fat
Chicken, Bacon & Swiss - Crispy	1	557	24	4	5	0	68	1684	51	2	33	3 1/2 starch, 3 lean meat, 3 fat

	Amount	Cal.	Fat (g)	% Cal. Fat	Sat. Fat (g)	Trans Fat (g)	Chol. (mg)	Sod. (mg)	Carb. (g)	Fiber (g)	Pro. (g)	Choices/Exchanges
Chicken, Bacon & Swiss - Grilled	1	443	17	3	4	0	77	1421	40	2	38	2 1/2 starch, 4 lean meat, 1 fat
✔ Popcorn Chicken	reg	363	16	4	3	0	54	930	27	2	24	2 starch, 3 lean meat, 1 1/2 fat
Popcorn Chicken	lg	529	24	4	4	0	79	1354	39	3	35	2 1/2 starch, 4 lean meat, 2 1/2 fat
Popcorn Chicken Shakers	1 srvg	582	24	4	4	0	79	2483	51	3	36	3 1/2 starch, 4 lean meat, 2 1/2 fat
BREAKFAST												
Bacon & Egg Croissant	1	337	22	6	10	0	187	651	23	1	11	1 1/2 starch, 1 high-fat meat, 2 fat
Bacon Biscuit	1	340	21	6	6	0	13	1028	29	1	9	2 starch, 3 1/2 fat
Bacon, Egg & Cheese Biscuit	1	461	28	5	8	0	169	1446	30	1	17	2 starch, 2 medium-fat meat, 4 fat

(Continued)

✔ = Healthiest Bets

BREAKFAST *(Continued)*	Amount	Cal.	Fat (g)	% Cal. Fat	Sat. Fat (g)	Trans Fat (g)	Chol. (mg)	Sod. (mg)	Carb. (g)	Fiber (g)	Pro. (g)	Choices/Exchanges
Bacon, Egg & Cheese Croissant	1	378	22	5	10	0	198	850	23	1	14	1 1/2 starch, 1 medium-fat meat, 3 fat
Bacon, Egg & Cheese Sourdough	1	437	16	3	5	0	174	1220	40	2	20	2 1/2 starch, 2 medium-fat meat, 1 1/2 fat
Bacon, Egg & Cheese Wrap	1	515	29	5	8	0.5	165	1367	50	2	16	3 1/2 starch, 1 medium-fat meat, 5 fat
Blueberry Muffin	1	320	12	3	2	0	20	190	49	1	4	3 1/2 starch, 2 1/2 fat
✔Breakfast Syrup	1 oz	78	0	0	0	0	0	25	20	0	0	1 carb
Chicken Biscuit	1	417	23	5	5	0	17	1240	39	1	15	2 1/2 starch, 1 lean meat, 4 fat
✔Croissant	1	190	10	5	6	0	30	190	21	1	3	1 starch, 2 fat
Egg & Cheese Sourdough	1	392	12	3	3	0	166	1058	40	2	17	2 1/2 starch, 1 medium-fat meat, 1 fat

	Amount											Exchanges/Choices
✔ French Toastix	1 order	312	13	4	2	0	0	492	44	1	6	3 starch, 3 fat
✔ Ham & Swiss Croissant	1	281	12	4	7	0	55	918	22	1	14	1 1/2 starch, 1 medium-fat meat, 1 fat
Ham Biscuit	1	323	17	5	4	0	15	1315	29	1	14	2 starch, 1 lean meat, 2 1/2 fat
Ham, Egg & Cheese Biscuit	1	444	24	5	6	0	171	1734	31	1	21	2 starch, 2 medium-fat meat, 2 1/2 fat
Ham, Egg & Cheese Croissant	1	361	18	4	9	0	200	1138	23	1	19	1 1/2 starch, 2 medium-fat meat, 1 1/2 fat
Ham, Egg, & Cheese Sourdough	1	442	14	3	4	0	180	1586	41	2	26	2 1/2 starch, 3 medium-fat meat, 1/2 fat
Ham, Egg, & Cheese Wrap	1	575	31	5	10	1	185	2005	51	2	25	3 1/2 starch, 2 medium-fat meat, 4 fat
Sausage & Egg Wrap	1	433	32	7	13	0	206	781	23	1	12	1 1/2 starch, 1 medium-fat meat, 5 1/2 fat

(Continued)

✔ = Healthiest Bets

BREAKFAST (Continued)	Amount	Cal.	Fat (g)	% Cal. Fat	Sat. Fat (g)	Trans Fat (g)	Chol. (mg)	Sod. (mg)	Carb. (g)	Fiber (g)	Pro. (g)	Choices/Exchanges
Sausage Biscuit	1	436	31	6	9	0	32	1160	28	1	10	2 starch, 1 medium-fat meat, 5 1/2 fat
Sausage Gravy Biscuit	1	961	68	6	14	0	12	3755	107	1	7	7 starch, 1 high-fat meat, 7 fat
Sausage Patty	1	210	20	9	7	0	40	480	0	0	6	1 high-fat meat, 2 1/2 fat
Sausage, Egg & Cheese Biscuit	1	557	38	6	11	0	187	1579	30	1	18	2 starch, 2 medium-fat meat, 6 fat
Sausage, Egg & Cheese Croissant	1	475	32	6	13	0	216	982	23	1	15	1 1/2 starch, 1 medium-fat meat, 5 fat
Sausage, Egg & Cheese Sourdough	1	556	28	5	9	0	197	1431	40	2	22	2 1/2 starch, 2 medium-fat meat, 3 1/2 fat
Sausage, Egg & Cheese Wrap	1	689	45	6	15	1	202	1849	50	2	21	3 1/2 starch, 2 medium-fat meat, 7 fat

CHICKEN DIPPING SAUCES

	Amount	Cal.	Fat (g)	% Cal. Fat	Sat. Fat (g)	Trans Fat (g)	Chol. (mg)	Sod. (mg)	Carb. (g)	Fiber (g)	Pro. (g)	Choices/Exchanges
✓ BBQ	1 oz	44	0	0	0	0	0	343	11	0	0	1/2 carb
✓ Buffalo	1 oz	10	1	9	0	0	0	790	2	0	0	Free
Honey Mustard	1 oz	129	12	8	2	0.25	9	151	6	0	0	1/2 carb, 2 1/2 fat

KID'S MENU

	Amount	Cal.	Fat (g)	% Cal. Fat	Sat. Fat (g)	Trans Fat (g)	Chol. (mg)	Sod. (mg)	Carb. (g)	Fiber (g)	Pro. (g)	Choices/Exchanges
✓ Fruit Cup	1	35	0	0	0	0	0	0	9	1	0	1 fruit
✓ Junior Roast Beef Sandwich	1	272	10	3	4	0	29	740	34	2	16	2 1/2 starch, 1 medium-fat meat, 1/2 fat
✓ Kid's Meal - Popcorn Chicken	1 srvg	272	12	4	2	0	41	698	20	1	18	1 1/2 starch, 2 lean meat, 1 fat
✓ Mini Ham & Cheese Sandwich	1	235	5	2	2	0	26	992	28	2	15	2 starch, 1 lean meat
✓ Mini Turkey & Cheese Sandwich	1	244	5	2	1	0	37	854	28	2	19	2 starch, 2 lean meat

(Continued)

✓ = Healthiest Bets

	Amount	Cal.	Fat (g)	% Cal. Fat	Sat. Fat (g)	Trans Fat (g)	Chol. (mg)	Sod. (mg)	Carb. (g)	Fiber (g)	Pro. (g)	Choices/Exchanges
MARKET FRESH SALADS												
Chicken Club Salad	1	425	22	5	7	0	180	894	26	4	28	1 starch, 3 veg, 4 lean meat, 2 1/2 fat
✓ Martha's Vineyard	1	273	9	3	4	0	61	609	25	4	22	1/2 starch, 3 veg, 3 lean meat
✓ Santa Fe Salad	1	415	17	4	5	0	55	806	37	6	25	1 1/2 starch, 3 veg, 3 lean meat, 1 1/2 fat
✓ Santa Fe Salad w/ Grilled Chicken	1	279	9	3	1	0	61	679	21	6	18	1/2 starch, 3 veg, 2 lean meat, 1/2 fat
MARKET FRESH SANDWICHES & WRAPS												
Corned Beef Reuben Sandwich	1	590	32	5	9	0.5	77	1685	55	3	32	3 1/2 starch, 3 medium-fat meat, 2 1/2 fat
Corned Reuben Wrap	1	560	29	5	8	0.5	77	1556	42	11	36	3 starch, 4 medium-fat meat, 1 fat

	Amount										Exchanges/Choices
Pecan Chicken Salad Sandwich	1	769	39	5	10	0	74	1240	79	9	30	5 1/2 starch, 2 lean meat, 5 1/2 fat
Pecan Chicken Salad Wrap	1	638	38	5	10	1	74	1199	48	8	30	3 starch, 3 medium-fat meat, 4 fat
Roast Ham & Swiss Sandwich	1	691	31	4	8	0.5	59	1952	75	5	33	5 starch, 3 lean meat, 4 fat
Roast Turkey & Bacon Sandwich	1	818	38	4	11	0.5	102	2146	75	5	46	5 starch, 4 lean meat, 4 1/2 fat
Roast Turkey & Swiss Sandwich	1	708	30	4	8	0.5	83	1677	74	5	41	5 starch, 4 lean meat, 3 fat
Roast Turkey Ranch & Bacon Wrap	1	683	37	5	11	1	102	2103	44	4	45	3 starch, 5 lean meat, 4 1/2 fat
Roast Turkey Reuben Sandwich	1	594	30	5	8	0.5	86	1318	56	3	40	3 1/2 starch, 4 lean meat, 2 1/2 fat
Roast Turkey Wrap	1	564	27	4	7	0	86	1189	43	11	44	3 starch, 5 lean meat, 2 fat

(Continued)

✓ = Healthiest Bets

MARKET FRESH SANDWICHES & WRAPS *(Continued)*	Amount	Cal.	Fat (g)	% Cal. Fat	Sat. Fat (g)	Trans Fat (g)	Chol. (mg)	Sod. (mg)	Carb. (g)	Fiber (g)	Pro. (g)	Choices/Exchanges
Southwest Chicken Wrap	1	563	30	5	9	1	77	1609	42	4	32	3 starch, 3 lean meat, 4 fat
Ultimate BLT Sandwich	1	779	45	5	11	0.5	51	1571	75	6	23	5 starch, 1 medium-fat meat, 7 1/2 fat
Ultimate BLT Wrap	1	648	44	6	11	1	51	1530	45	6	23	3 starch, 2 medium-fat meat, 6 1/2 fat

MARKET SALAD DRESSINGS & TOPPINGS

	Amount	Cal.	Fat (g)	% Cal. Fat	Sat. Fat (g)	Trans Fat (g)	Chol. (mg)	Sod. (mg)	Carb. (g)	Fiber (g)	Pro. (g)	Choices/Exchanges
Buttermilk Ranch Dressing	2 oz	325	34	9	5	0.5	28	657	4	0	1	1/2 carb, 7 fat
✓ Garlic & Cheese Croutons	1 srvg	77	5	6	1	0	1	116	7	0	2	1/2 starch, 1 fat
Light Buttermilk Ranch Dressing	2 oz	112	6	5	1	0	1	472	12	1	1	1 carb, 1 fat
Raspberry Vinaigrette	2 oz	194	14	6	2	0	0	387	18	0	0	1 carb, 3 fat
Santa Fe Ranch Dressing	2 oz	296	31	9	5	0	21	692	4	0	1	1/2 carb, 6 fat

Item	Amount	Cal.	Fat (g)	% Cal. Fat	Sat. Fat (g)	Trans Fat (g)	Chol. (mg)	Sod. (mg)	Carb. (g)	Fiber (g)	Pro. (g)	Servings/Exchanges
✓ Seasoned Crouton Strips	1 srvg	71	3	38	0	0	0	25	9	1	1	1/2 starch, 1/2 fat
Sliced Almonds	1 srvg	81	8	89	1	0	0	0	2	1	4	2 fat
ROAST BEEF SANDWICHES & MELTS												
✓ Arby's Melt	1	302	12	36	4	0	30	921	36	2	16	2 1/2 starch, 1 medium-fat meat, 1 fat
✓ Arby's Sauce	.5 oz	15	0	0	0	0	0	177	4	0	0	Free
Bacon Beef 'n Cheddar Sandwich	1	521	27	47	9	1.5	64	1573	45	2	27	3 starch, 3 medium-fat meat, 3 fat
BBQ Beef 'n Jack	1	360	16	40	5	0.5	37	1175	42	2	19	3 starch, 2 medium-fat meat, 1 fat
Beef 'n Cheddar Sandwich	1	445	21	42	6	1.5	51	1274	44	2	22	3 starch, 2 medium-fat meat, 2 1/2 fat
Ham & Swiss Melt Sandwich	1	268	5	17	2	0	25	1042	35	1	17	2 1/2 starch, 1 lean meat

(Continued)

✓ = Healthiest Bets

ROAST BEEF SANDWICHES & MELTS (Continued)	Amount	Cal.	Fat (g)	% Cal. Fat	Sat. Fat (g)	Trans Fat (g)	Chol. (mg)	Sod. (mg)	Carb. (g)	Fiber (g)	Pro. (g)	Choices/Exchanges
Horsey Sauce	.5 oz	62	5	7	1	0	5	173	3	0	0	1 fat
✔ Junior Roast Beef Sandwich	1	272	10	3	4	0	29	740	34	2	16	2 1/2 starch, 1 medium-fat meat, 1/2 fat
Roast Beef Sandwich	med	415	21	5	9	1	73	1379	34	2	31	2 1/2 starch, 3 medium-fat meat, 1/2 fat
Roast Beef Sandwich	super	398	19	4	6	0.5	44	1060	40	2	21	2 1/2 starch, 2 medium-fat meat, 2 fat
✔ Roast Beef Sandwich	reg	320	14	4	5	0.5	44	953	34	2	21	2 1/2 starch, 2 medium-fat meat, 1 fat
Roast Beef Sandwich	lg	547	28	5	12	1.5	102	1869	41	3	42	2 1/2 starch, 5 medium-fat meat, 1/2 fat
Sourdough Ham Melt	1	380	13	3	3	0	31	1280	39	2	19	2 1/2 starch, 2 lean meat, 1 1/2 fat
Sourdough Roast Beef Melt	1	355	14	4	5	1	30	1047	40	2	18	2 1/2 starch, 1 medium-fat meat, 1 1/2 fat

✔ Spicy Three Pepper Sauce	.5 oz	22	1	4	0	0	0	140	3	0	0	1/2 fat
✔ Swiss Melt	1	303	12	4	4	1	29	919	37	2	16	2 1/2 starch, 1 medium-fat meat, 1 fat

SHAKES & DESSERTS

Apple Turnover	1	337	16	4	5	6.5	0	201	65	2	4	4 starch, 1 1/2 fat
Berry Delight Swirl Shake	1	651	16	2	9	0.5	39	439	112	0	15	7 starch, 2 fat
Cherry Turnover	1	337	15	4	5	6	0	201	65	2	4	4 starch, 2 fat
✔ Chocolate Chip Cookie	1	202	10	4	4	2	15	213	26	1	2	2 starch, 2 fat
Chocolate Shake	reg	507	13	2	8	0	34	357	83	0	13	6 starch, 2 1/2 fat
Chocolate Shake	lg	660	17	2	10	0.5	43	455	110	1	17	7 starch, 2 fat
Chocolate Turnover	1	400	25	6	7	7	0	190	37	4	6	2 starch, 5 fat
Jamocha Shake	reg	498	13	2	8	0	34	393	81	0	13	5 starch, 2 fat
Jamocha Shake	lg	647	17	2	10	0.5	43	509	107	1	17	7 starch, 2 1/2 fat

(Continued)

✔ = Healthiest Bets

SHAKES & DESSERTS (Continued)	Amount	Cal.	Fat (g)	% Cal. Fat	Sat. Fat (g)	Trans Fat (g)	Chol. (mg)	Sod. (mg)	Carb. (g)	Fiber (g)	Pro. (g)	Choices/Exchanges
Strawberry Shake	reg	498	13	2	8	0	34	363	81	0	13	5 starch, 1 1/2 fat
Strawberry Shake	lg	646	17	2	10	0.5	43	464	107	1	16	7 starch, 2 1/2 fat
Vanilla Shake	reg	437	13	3	8	0	34	350	66	0	13	4 starch, 2 1/2 fat
Vanilla Shake	lg	555	17	3	10	0.5	43	445	83	0	16	6 starch, 3 1/2 fat
SIDES & SIDEKICKERS												
Bronco Berry Dipping Sauce	2 oz	122	0	0	0	0	0	36	30	0	0	2 carb
✓Cheddar Cheese Sauce	side portion	30	2	6	1	0.5	1	181	2	0	0	1 fat
Cheddar Fries	med	465	28	5	6	2	2	1311	51	5	6	3 starch, 5 fat
Cool Ranch Sour Cream Dipping Sauce	1.5 oz	158	16	9	4	0	0	277	2	0	1	3 fat
Curly Fries	sm	338	20	5	4	0	0	791	39	4	4	3 starch, 3 1/2 fat

Curly Fries	med	397	24	5	4	0	0	928	45	4	5	3 starch, 4 fat
Curly Fries	lg	631	37	5	7	1	0	1476	73	7	8	5 starch, 6 fat
Jalapeño Bites, med	5	305	21	6	9	1	28	526	29	2	5	2 starch, 4 fat
Jalapeño Bites, lg	10	611	43	6	18	1.5	56	1052	58	4	11	4 starch, 7 1/2 fat
Loaded Potato Bites, med	5	353	22	6	7	0.5	13	800	27	2	11	2 starch, 4 1/2 fat
Loaded Potato Bites, lg	10	707	44	6	14	1.5	27	1601	54	5	23	4 starch, 9 fat
✔Marinara Sauce	1.5 oz	30	2	6	0	0	0	0	4	1	1	Free
Mozzarella Sticks, med	4	426	28	6	13	1	45	1370	38	2	18	2 1/2 starch, 1 medium-fat meat, 3 fat
Mozzarella Sticks, lg	8	849	56	6	26	2	90	2730	75	4	36	5 starch, 11 fat
Onion Petals	reg	331	23	6	4	0	1	332	35	2	4	2 starch, 4 fat
Onion Petals	lg	828	57	6	9	1	2	831	88	5	10	6 starch, 8 fat
Potato Cakes	2	246	18	7	4	1	0	391	26	2	2	2 starch, 3 fat

(Continued)

✔ = Healthiest Bets

SIDES & SIDEKICKERS (Continued)	Amount	Cal.	Fat (g)	% Cal. Fat	Sat. Fat (g)	Trans Fat (g)	Chol. (mg)	Sod. (mg)	Carb. (g)	Fiber (g)	Pro. (g)	Choices/Exchanges
Potato Cakes	3	369	28	7	5	1.5	0	587	39	3	3	3 starch, 4 fat
Tangy Southwest Sauce	2 oz	333	35	9	5	0.5	29	371	5	0	1	7 fat
T.J. CINNAMONS												
Chocolate Twist	1	250	12	4	4	0	5	110	34	2	4	2 1/2 carb, 2 1/2 fat
Cinnamon Twist	1	260	14	5	5	4	5	190	33	1	3	2 carb, 3 fat
Original Gourmet Cinnamon Roll	1	507	10	2	4	0	7	373	73	4	10	5 carb, 2 fat
Pecan Sticky Bun	1	688	22	3	5	0	7	420	91	5	12	6 carb, 4 1/2 fat
T.J. Cinnamon Mocha Chill	1	306	7	2	4	0	29	214	48	1	11	3 carb, 1 1/2 fat
T.J. Icing	1 oz	117	5	4	2	1	8	50	18	0	1	1 carb, 1 fat
TOASTED SUBS												
Classic Italian	1	787	39	4	9	0.5	81	1642	67	3	33	4 1/2 starch, 3 medium-fat meat, 5 fat

French Dip & Swiss	1	622	20	3	7	1.5	79	3397	68	3	37	4 1/2 starch, 3 medium-fat meat, 1/2 fat
Philly Beef	1	739	37	5	9	1	85	1881	64	3	32	4 1/2 starch, 3 medium-fat meat, 4 1/2 fat
Turkey Bacon	1	619	18	3	4	0	82	2052	65	3	42	4 1/2 starch, 4 medium-fat meat

✓ = Healthiest Bets

Baskin Robbins
(www.baskinrobbins.com)

Baskin Robbins

	Amount	Cal.	Fat (g)	% Cal. Fat	Sat. Fat (g)	Trans Fat (g)	Chol. (mg)	Sod. (mg)	Carb. (g)	Fiber (g)	Pro. (g)	Choices/Exchanges
BEVERAGES: CAPPUCCINO BLAST												
Caramel	16 oz.	480	16	3	10	0	60	300	81	0	7	5 1/2 carb, 2 fat
Caramel	24 oz.	720	24	3	15	0.5	90	440	121	0	10	8 carb, 4 fat
Caramel	32 oz.	1000	30	3	19	1	115	650	173	0	13	11 1/2 carb, 5 fat
Low Fat	16 oz.	220	2	1	1.5	0	10	115	45	0	6	3 carb
Mocha	16 oz.	380	12	3	7	0	45	85	64	0	5	4 1/2 carb, 2 fat
Mocha	24 oz.	540	18	3	12	0	70	140	87	0	8	6 carb, 3 fat
Mocha	32 oz.	750	23	3	15	0	90	170	128	0	11	8 1/2 carb, 4 fat
Mocha w/Whipped Cream	16 oz.	370	13	3	8	0	50	100	58	0	6	4 carb, 2 fat
Mocha w/Whipped Cream	24 oz.	620	21	3	13	0	80	160	100	0	9	6 1/2 carb, 3 fat

✓ = Healthiest Bets

(Continued)

BEVERAGES: CAPPUCCINO BLAST *(Continued)*	Amount	Cal.	Fat (g)	% Cal. Fat	Sat. Fat (g)	Trans Fat (g)	Chol. (mg)	Sod. (mg)	Carb. (g)	Fiber (g)	Pro. (g)	Choices/Exchanges
Mocha w/ Whipped Cream	32 oz.	790	25	3	16	0	100	190	136	0	11	9 carb, 4 fat
Nonfat	16 oz.	210	0	0	0	0	5	120	45	0	7	3 carb
Nonfat	24 oz.	340	0	0	0	0	5	190	78	0	11	5 carb
Nonfat	32 oz.	440	0.5	0	0	0	5	240	102	1	14	7 carb
Original	16 oz.	300	12	4	7	0	45	95	43	0	6	3 carb, 2 fat
Original	24 oz.	460	19	4	12	0	75	150	66	0	9	4 1/2 carb, 3 fat
Original	32 oz.	620	24	3	15	0	95	200	94	0	12	6 1/2 carb, 4 fat
w/ Whipped Cream	16 oz.	330	14	4	9	0	55	110	48	0	6	3 carb, 2 fat
w/ Whipped Cream	24 oz.	480	21	4	13	0	80	160	67	0	9	4 1/2 carb, 3 fat
w/ Whipped Cream	32 oz.	660	28	4	17	0	105	220	97	0	12	6 1/2 carb, 4 fat
BEVERAGES: FREEZES												
w/ Orange Sherbet	16 oz.	370	4	1	2.5	0	15	120	82	0	3	5 1/2 carb, 1/2 fat

(Continued)

	Amount	Cal.	Fat (g)	% Cal. Fat	Sat. Fat (g)	Trans Fat (g)	Chol. (mg)	Sod. (mg)	Carb. (g)	Fiber (g)	Pro. (g)	Servings/Exchanges
w/ Orange Sherbet	23 oz.	510	5	1	3.5	0	20	160	112	1	3	7 1/2 carb, 1/2 fat
w/ Orange Sherbet	33 oz.	740	8	1	5	0	30	240	164	1	5	11 carb, 1 fat
BEVERAGES: FRUIT BLAST												
Berry Pomegranate	16 oz.	370	0	0	0	0	0	15	93	1	0	6 carb
Berry Pomegranate	24 oz.	510	0	0	0	0	0	20	128	1	1	8 1/2 carb
Berry Pomegranate	32 oz.	740	0	0	0	0	0	30	186	1	1	12 1/2 carb
Peach Passion	16 oz.	270	0	0	0	0	0	10	68	2	1	4 1/2 carb
Peach Passion	24 oz.	370	0.5	1	0	0	0	10	94	3	2	6 1/2 carb
Peach Passion	32 oz.	500	1	2	0	0	0	15	136	4	3	9 carb
Strawberry Citrus	16 oz.	350	1	0	0	0	0	10	89	3	1	6 carb
Strawberry Citrus	24 oz.	480	1	0	0	0	0	15	122	4	2	8 carb
Strawberry Citrus	32 oz.	700	1.5	0	0	0	0	20	178	6	3	12 carb
Wild Mango	16 oz.	340	1	0	0	0	0	10	84	2	1	5 1/2 carb

✓ = Healthiest Bets

BEVERAGES: FRUIT BLAST (Continued)	Amount	Cal.	Fat (g)	% Cal. Fat	Sat. Fat (g)	Trans Fat (g)	Chol. (mg)	Sod. (mg)	Carb. (g)	Fiber (g)	Pro. (g)	Choices/Exchanges
Wild Mango	24 oz.	470	1.5	0	0	0	0	15	116	2	1	7 1/2 carb
Wild Mango	32 oz.	690	2	0	0	0	0	20	169	3	1	11 1/2 carb
BEVERAGES: FRUIT BLAST SMOOTHIE												
Berry Pomegranate Banana	16 oz.	510	0.5	0	0	0	0	80	125	2	5	8 1/2 carb
Berry Pomegranate Banana	24 oz.	710	1	0	0	0	5	125	172	3	7	11 1/2 carb
Berry Pomegranate Banana	32 oz.	1020	1.5	0	0.5	0	5	160	250	5	9	16 1/2 carb
Mango	16 oz.	440	1.5	0	0	0	0	75	104	2	4	7 carb
Mango	24 oz.	620	2	0	0	0	5	120	148	3	7	10 carb
Mango	32 oz.	870	3	0	0	0	5	150	209	4	8	14 carb
Peach Passion	16 oz.	420	1	0	0	0	0	70	102	4	6	7 carb
Peach Passion	24 oz.	540	1	0	0	0	5	110	131	5	8	8 1/2 carb
Peach Passion	32 oz.	830	1.5	0	0.5	0	5	140	204	8	11	13 1/2 carb

	Amount	Cal.	Fat (g)	% Cal. Fat	Sat. Fat (g)	Trans Fat (g)	Chol. (mg)	Sod. (mg)	Carb. (g)	Fiber (g)	Prot. (g)	Choices/Exchanges
Strawberry Banana	16 oz.	490	1.5	0	0	0	0	75	121	5	5	8 carb
Strawberry Banana	24 oz.	730	2	0	0		5	120	178	7	9	12 carb
Strawberry Banana	32 oz.	980	2.5	0	0.5		5	150	242	9	11	16 carb
BEVERAGES: ICE CREAM FLOATS												
w/Vanilla Ice Cream & Root Beer	17 oz.	470	20	4	13	0.5	80	130	69	0	6	4 1/2 carb, 3 fat
w/Vanilla Ice Cream & Root Beer	24 oz.	680	30	4	19	1	120	190	99	0	8	6 1/2 carb, 5 fat
w/Vanilla Ice Cream & Root Beer	34 oz.	940	40	4	25	1.5	155	260	138	0	11	9 carb, 7 fat
BEVERAGES: ICE CREAM SODAS												
w/Vanilla Ice Cream	14 oz.	480	20	4	13	0.5	80	130	69	0	6	4 1/2 carb, 3 fat
w/Vanilla Ice Cream	21 oz.	720	30	4	19	1	120	190	103	0	8	7 carb, 5 fat
w/Vanilla Ice Cream	29 oz.	960	40	4	25	1.5	155	260	138	0	11	9 carb, 7 fat

✔ = Healthiest Bets

(Continued)

	Amount	Cal.	Fat (g)	% Cal. Fat	Sat. Fat (g)	Trans Fat (g)	Chol. (mg)	Sod. (mg)	Carb. (g)	Fiber (g)	Pro. (g)	Choices/Exchanges
BEVERAGES: PREMIUM SHAKES												
Chocolate Oreo	16 oz.	1040	56	5	26	1.5	85	630	126	5	16	8 1/2 carb, 9 fat
Chocolate Oreo	24 oz.	1490	79	5	36	1.5	110	950	186	7	23	12 1/2 carb, 14 fat
Chocolate Oreo	32 oz.	2600	135	5	59	2.5	185	1770	333	13	38	22 carb, 24 fat
Heath	16 oz.	990	46	4	28	1	130	670	129	1	16	8 1/2 carb, 8 fat
Heath	24 oz.	1420	67	4	40	1.5	180	960	184	1	23	12 1/2 carb, 11 fat
Heath	32 oz.	2310	108	4	64	2.5	295	1560	303	2	35	20 carb, 18 fat
Jamoca Oreo	16 oz.	790	31	4	18	1	90	560	117	1	14	8 carb, 5 fat
Jamoca Oreo	24 oz.	1170	44	3	25	1	120	890	177	2	21	12 carb, 7 fat
Jamoca Oreo	32 oz.	1890	73	3	41	2	205	1380	283	4	32	19 carb, 12 fat
Oreo Cookies n Cream	16 oz.	990	46	4	25	1	110	660	132	2	16	9 carb, 7 fat
Oreo Cookies n Cream	24 oz.	1410	62	4	33	1.5	145	940	195	4	23	13 carb, 11 fat

Oreo Cookies n Cream	32 oz.	2210	100	4	54	2	245	1400	302	5	35	20 carb, 17 fat
Reeses Peanut Butter Cup	16 oz.	1010	62	6	27	1	110	560	93	4	24	6 carb, 12 fat
Reeses Peanut Butter Cup	24 oz.	1430	93	6	36	1	140	830	122	6	36	8 carb, 18 fat
Reeses Peanut Butter Cup	32 oz.	2320	150	6	60	2	235	1320	204	10	56	13 1/2 carb, 27 fat
York Peppermint Pattie	16 oz.	960	44	4	25	1	100	290	132	2	14	9 carb, 7 fat
York Peppermint Pattie	24 oz.	1390	62	4	35	1	135	440	195	3	20	13 carb, 11 fat
York Peppermint Pattie	32 oz.	2210	103	4	57	2	225	680	304	6	31	20 1/2 carb, 17 fat

BEVERAGES: SHAKES

Chocolate Chip	16 oz.	540	21	4	14	0.5	65	300	77	1	15	5 carb, 3 fat
Chocolate Chip	24 oz.	750	28	3	18	1	85	410	106	2	21	7 carb, 5 fat
Chocolate Chip	32 oz.	1220	48	4	31	1.5	145	680	170	3	34	11 1/2 carb, 8 fat
Chocolate w/ Chocolate Ice Cream	16 oz.	620	30	4	18	1	105	300	81	1	15	5 1/2 carb, 5 fat

✔ = Healthiest Bets

(Continued)

BEVERAGES: SHAKES *(Continued)*	Amount	Cal.	Fat (g)	% Cal. Fat	Sat. Fat (g)	Trans Fat (g)	Chol. (mg)	Sod. (mg)	Carb. (g)	Fiber (g)	Pro. (g)	Choices/Exchanges
Chocolate w/ Chocolate Ice Cream	24 oz.	990	40	4	25	1	135	440	149	1	20	10 carb, 6 fat
Chocolate w/ Chocolate Ice Cream	32 oz.	1290	58	4	36	0	200	630	176	1	28	11 1/2 carb, 10 fat
Chocolate w/ Vanilla Ice Cream	16 oz.	690	33	4	21	0	130	210	85	0	13	5 1/2 carb, 5 fat
Chocolate w/ Vanilla Ice Cream	24 oz.	1000	45	4	28	0	175	290	133	0	19	9 carb, 7 fat
Chocolate w/ Vanilla Ice Cream	32 oz.	1300	66	5	42	0	260	420	152	0	27	10 carb, 11 fat
Mint Chocolate Chip	16 oz.	760	36	4	24	0	115	320	94	1	16	6 1/2 carb, 6 fat
Mint Chocolate Chip	24 oz.	970	47	4	31	0	155	410	116	2	21	7 1/2 carb, 8 fat
Mint Chocolate Chip	32 oz.	1520	72	4	47	0	225	630	189	3	31	12 1/2 carb, 13 fat

	Amount	Cal	Fat (g)	% Cal. Fat	Sat. Fat (g)	Trans Fat (g)	Chol. (mg)	Sod. (mg)	Carb. (g)	Fiber (g)	Pro. (g)	Choices/Exchanges
Strawberry w/ Very Berry Strawberry Ice Cream	16 oz.	470	14	3	9	0	50	270	75	1	13	5 carb, 2 fat
Strawberry w/ Very Berry Strawberry Ice Cream	24 oz.	650	19	3	12	0.5	70	370	104	1	18	7 carb, 3 fat
Strawberry w/ Very Berry Strawberry Ice Cream	32 oz.	1120	46	4	29	1.5	185	440	154	2	24	10 1/2 carb, 7 fat
Vanilla	16 oz.	680	33	4	21	0	130	380	81	0	13	5 1/2 carb, 6 fat
Vanilla	24 oz.	980	45	4	28	0	175	640	125	0	19	8 1/2 carb, 7 fat
Vanilla	32 oz.	1290	66	5	42	0	260	650	147	0	27	10 carb, 11 fat
CAKES: ROLL ICE CREAM CAKES												
Chocolate Chip Ice Cream/Chocolate	1 slice	290	15	5	6	0	40	340	41	2	4	2 1/2 carb, 2 fat
Mint Chocolate Chip Ice Cream/Chocolate	1 slice	290	14	4	6	0	45	240	36	2	5	2 1/2 carb, 3 fat
Vanilla Ice Cream/Chocolate	1 slice	270	14	5	4	0	45	340	39	2	4	2 1/2 carb, 2 fat

✔ = Healthiest Bets

(Continued)

	Amount	Cal.	Fat (g)	% Cal. Fat	Sat. Fat (g)	Trans Fat (g)	Chol. (mg)	Sod. (mg)	Carb. (g)	Fiber (g)	Pro. (g)	Choices/Exchanges
CAKES: ROUND ICE CREAM CAKES												
Chocolate Chip Cookie Dough Ice Cream/ Devils Food 6"	1 slice	460	23	5	11	0	65	380	59	1	7	4 carb, 4 fat
Chocolate Chip Ice Cream/ Devils Food 9"	1 slice	410	23	5	11	0	70	320	51	2	6	3 1/2 carb, 4 fat
Oreo Cookies n Cream Ice Cream/ Devils Food 6"	1 slice	440	23	5	10	0	65	400	56	1	7	3 1/2 carb, 4 fat
Oreo Cookies n Cream Ice Cream/ Devils Food 9"	1 slice	430	23	5	10	0.5	65	390	55	1	7	3 1/2 carb, 4 fat
Pralines n Cream Ice Cream/ White Sponge 9"	1 slice	430	20	4	8	0	50	380	65	1	6	4 1/2 carb, 3 fat
Vanilla & Chocolate Ice Cream/ Fudge Crunch 9"	1 slice	340	18	5	12	1	45	170	41	1	5	2 1/2 carb, 3 fat

CAKES: SHEET ICE CREAM CAKES

Chocolate Chip Ice Cream/Devils Food	1 slice	330	18	5	8	0	55	240	41	1	5	2 1/2 carb, 3 fat
Mint Chocolate Chip Ice Cream/Devils Food	1 slice	330	18	5	8	0	55	240	41	1	5	2 1/2 carb, 3 fat
Oreo Cookies n Cream Ice Cream/White Sponge	1 slice	350	16	4	7	0	45	270	47	1	5	3 carb, 3 fat
Pralines n Cream Ice Cream/White Sponge	1 slice	360	16	4	6	0	40	280	49	1	5	3 1/2 carb, 3 fat
Vanilla & Chocolate Ice Cream/Fudge Crunch	1 slice	330	18	5	12	1	45	160	40	1	5	2 1/2 carb, 3 fat
Vanilla Ice Cream/Devils Food	1 slice	340	19	5	9	0	60	220	39	1	5	2 1/2 carb, 4 fat
Very Berry Strawberry Ice Cream/White Sponge	1 slice	310	13	4	6	0	40	210	44	1	4	3 carb, 2 fat

(Continued)

✓ = Healthiest Bets

	Amount	Cal.	Fat (g)	% Cal. Fat	Sat. Fat (g)	Trans Fat (g)	Chol. (mg)	Sod. (mg)	Carb. (g)	Fiber (g)	Pro. (g)	Choices/Exchanges
CAKES: SPECIALTY ICE CREAM CAKES												
Chocolate Chip Ice Cream/ Devils Food Heart	1 slice	330	18	5	8	0	55	240	40	1	5	2 1/2 carb, 3 fat
Vanilla Ice Cream/ Devils Food Heart	1 slice	340	19	5	9	0	60	220	39	1	5	2 1/2 carb, 3 fat
GRAB-N-GO: FRUIT BLAST BARS												
✓Blue Raspberry	1 bar	50	0	0	0	0	0	0	14	0	0	1 carb
✓Mango	1 bar	50	0	0	0	0	0	0	14	0	0	1 carb
✓Strawberry	1 bar	50	0	0	0	0	0	0	13	0	0	1 carb
GRAB-N-GO: PRE-PACKED ICE CREAM												
✓Chocolate Chip Ice Cream Quart	1/2 cup	170	10	5	6	0	35	55	18	0	3	1 carb, 2 fat

✔ Chocolate Cookie Dough Ice Cream Quart	1/2 cup	200	10	5	6	0	30	85	23	0	3	3 1/2 carb, 2 fat
✔ Chocolate Ice Cream Quart	1/2 cup	170	9	5	6	0	30	85	21	1	3	1 1/2 carb, 2 fat
✔ Chocolate Oreo Ice Cream Quart	1/2 cup	200	11	5	5	0	25	110	24	1	3	1 1/2 carb, 2 fat
✔ Gold Medal Ribbon Ice Cream Quart	1/2 cup	170	8	4	5	0	30	105	22	0	3	1 1/2 carb, 1 1/2 fat
✔ Heath Ice Cream Quart	1/2 cup	200	10	5	6	0	30	115	25	0	3	1 1/2 carb, 2 fat
✔ Jamoca Almond Fudge Ice Cream Quart	1/2 cup	180	10	5	5	0	30	55	21	1	4	1 1/2 carb, 2 fat
✔ Love Potion #31 Ice Cream Quart	1/2 cup	180	9	5	6	0	30	55	22	1	3	1 1/2 carb, 2 fat
✔ Mint Chocolate Chip Ice Cream Quart	1/2 cup	170	10	5	6	0	35	55	18	0	3	1 carb, 2 fat
Old Fashioned Butter Pecan Ice Cream Quart	1/2 cup	180	12	6	6	0	35	70	16	1	3	1 carb, 2 1/2 fat

✔ = Healthiest Bets

(Continued)

GRAB-N-GO: PRE-PACKED ICE CREAM *(Continued)*	Amount	Cal.	Fat (g)	% Cal. Fat	Sat. Fat (g)	Trans Fat (g)	Chol. (mg)	Sod. (mg)	Carb. (g)	Fiber (g)	Pro. (g)	Choices/Exchanges
✔Oreo Cookies n Cream Ice Cream Quart	1/2 cup	180	10	5	6	0	30	100	21	0	3	1 1/2 carb, 2 fat
Peanut Butter n Chocolate Ice Cream Quart	1/2 cup	200	13	6	6	0	30	115	20	1	5	1 1/2 carb, 2 1/2 fat
✔Pralines n Cream Ice Cream Quart	1/2 cup	190	9	4	5	0	30	125	24	0	3	1 1/2 carb, 2 fat
✔Rainbow Sherbet Quart	1/2 cup	120	2	2	1	0	5	30	26	0	1	1 1/2 carb, 1/2 fat
Reeses Peanut Butter Cup Ice Cream Quart	1/2 cup	190	11	5	6	0	30	85	20	0	4	1 1/2 carb, 2 fat
✔Rocky Road Ice Cream Quart	1/2 cup	190	10	5	5	0	30	85	23	1	4	1 1/2 carb, 2 fat
✔Vanilla Ice Cream Quart	1/2 cup	170	10	5	7	0	40	45	17	0	3	1 carb, 2 fat
✔Very Berry Strawberry Ice Cream Quart	1/2 cup	140	7	5	4.5	0	25	45	18	0	2	1 carb, 1 1/2 fat

GRAB-N-GO: SUNDAE CUPS

Oreo	1 cup	330	15	4	7	0	40	190	45	0	4	3 carb, 2 fat
Pralines n Cream	1 cup	330	16	4	8	0	45	170	43	1	4	3 carb, 3 fat
Reeses Peanut Butter Cup	1 cup	390	24	6	9	0	40	190	36	2	8	2 1/2 carb, 5 fat

ICE CREAM: CLASSIC FLAVORS

Cherries Jubilee	1 scoop	240	12	5	7	0	45	80	30	1	4	2 carb, 2 1/2 fat
Chocolate	1 scoop	260	14	5	9	0	50	130	33	0	5	2 carb, 2 1/2 fat
Chocolate Chip	1 scoop	270	16	5	10	0	55	95	28	1	5	2 carb, 3 fat
Chocolate Chip Cookie Dough	1 scoop	290	15	5	9	1	55	130	36	1	5	2 1/2 carb, 3 fat
Chocolate Fudge	1 scoop	270	15	5	10	0	50	140	35	0	4	2 carb, 3 fat
French Vanilla	1 scoop	280	18	6	11	0.5	120	85	26	0	4	1 1/2 carb, 3 1/2 fat
Gold Medal Ribbon	1 scoop	260	13	5	8	0	45	150	34	0	5	2 1/2 carb, 2 fat
Heath	1 scoop	300	15	5	9	0	45	180	38	0	5	2 1/2 carb, 2 1/2 fat

✔ = Healthiest Bets

(Continued)

ICE CREAM: CLASSIC FLAVORS *(Continued)*	Amount	Cal.	Fat (g)	% Cal. Fat	Sat. Fat (g)	Trans Fat (g)	Chol. (mg)	Sod. (mg)	Carb. (g)	Fiber (g)	Pro. (g)	Choices/Exchanges
Jamoca	1 scoop	240	13	5	9	0	55	90	26	0	5	1 1/2 carb, 2 1/2 fat
Jamoca Almond Fudge	1 scoop	270	15	5	7	0	40	80	31	1	6	2 carb, 2 1/2 fat
Mint Chocolate Chip	1 scoop	270	16	5	10	0	55	95	28	1	5	2 carb, 3 fat
Nutty Coconut	1 scoop	300	20	6	9	0	45	90	28	1	6	2 carb, 4 fat
Old Fashioned Butter Pecan	1 scoop	280	18	6	9	0	50	95	24	1	5	1 1/2 carb, 3 1/2 fat
Peanut Butter n Chocolate	1 scoop	320	20	6	9	0	45	180	31	1	7	2 carb, 4 fat
Pistachio Almond	1 scoop	290	19	6	9	0	50	85	25	1	7	1 1/2 carb, 4 fat
Pralines n Cream	1 scoop	270	14	5	8	0	45	170	34	0	4	2 1/2 carb, 2 1/2 fat
Reeses Peanut Butter Cup	1 scoop	300	18	5	10	0	50	130	31	0	6	2 carb, 3 fat
Rocky Road	1 scoop	290	15	5	8	0	45	120	36	1	5	2 1/2 carb, 2 1/2 fat
Vanilla	1 scoop	260	16	6	10	0.5	65	70	26	0	4	1 1/2 carb, 3 fat

	Serving	Cal									
✔ Very Berry Strawberry	1 scoop	220	11	5	7	0	40	70	28	0	4	2 carb, 1 1/2 fat
World Class Chocolate	1 scoop	280	16	11		0	45	95	31	0	5	2 carb, 3 fat

ICE CREAM: CONES

	Serving	Cal									
✔ Cake	1 cone	25	0	0	0	0	0	15	5	0	0	1/2 carb
✔ Sugar	1 cone	45	1	2	0	0	0	35	9	0	1	1/2 carb
Waffle	1 cone	160	4	2	1	0	10	5	28	0	2	2 carb, 1 fat

ICE CREAM: FLAVORS OF THE MONTH

	Serving	Cal									
Chocolate Oreo	1 scoop	360	20	5	8	0	35	210	44	2	5	3 carb, 3 fat
Jamoca Oreo	1 scoop	270	12	4	7	0	40	135	36	1	4	2 1/2 carb, 2 1/2 fat
Oreo Cookies n Cream	1 scoop	280	15	5	9	0	50	150	32	1	5	2 carb, 3 fat

ICE CREAM: LIGHTER SIDE

	Serving	Cal									
✔ Berries n Banana w/o Sugar	1 scoop	110	2	2	1	n/a	125	125	25	1	5	1 1/2 carb
Caramel Turtle w/o Sugar	1 scoop	160	4	2	3	0	10	170	37	0	5	2 1/2 carb, 1/2 fat

✔ = Healthiest Bets

(Continued)

ICE CREAM: LIGHTER SIDE *(Continued)*	Amount	Cal.	Fat (g)	% Cal. Fat	Sat. Fat (g)	Trans Fat (g)	Chol. (mg)	Sod. (mg)	Carb. (g)	Fiber (g)	Pro. (g)	Choices/Exchanges
✓Chocolate Chocolate Chip w/o Sugar	1 scoop	150	5	3	3.5	0	10	140	31	1	6	2 carb, 1/2 fat
✓Espresso n Cream	1 scoop	180	4	2	1.5	0	10	120	32	1	5	2 carb, 1 fat
✓Lemon Sorbet	1 scoop	130	0	0	0	0	0	15	33	0	0	2 carb
✓Lime Daiquiri Ice	1 scoop	130	0	0	0	0	0	15	33	0	0	2 carb
Maui Brownie Madness Frozen Yogurt	1 scoop	210	4	2	1.5	n/a	10	135	40	2	6	2 1/2 carb, 1/2 fat
Orange Sherbet	1 scoop	160	2	1	1.5	0	10	40	34	0	1	2 1/2 carb, 1/2 fat
✓Pineapple Coconut Low Fat w/o Sugar	1 scoop	120	2	2	1.5	0	10	140	27	0	5	2 carb
Rainbow Sherbet	1 scoop	160	2	1	1.5	0	10	40	34	0	1	2 1/2 carb
Raspberry Cheese Louise Frozen Yogurt	1 scoop	190	3.5	2	2.5	0	10	150	35	1	5	2 1/2 carb, 1/2 fat

Red Raspberry Sherbet	1 scoop	160	2	1	1	0	10	40	35	1	2	2 1/2 carb
Rock n Pop Swirl Sherbet	1 scoop	190	4	2	3	0	10	45	37	0	1	2 1/2 carb, 1/2 fat
✔ Splish Splash Sherbet/Ice Swirl	1 scoop	140	1	1	0.5	0	5	25	33	0	1	2 carb
✔ Strawberry Sorbet	1 scoop	130	0	0	0	0	0	10	34	0	0	2 carb
✔ Tin Roof Sundae w/o Sugar	1 scoop	150	4	2	2	0	10	160	33	1	5	2 carb
Tropical Ice	1 scoop	140	0	0	0	0	0	15	35	0	0	2 1/2 carb
✔ Vanilla Nonfat Frozen Yogurt	1 scoop	150	0	0	0	0	5	105	32	0	6	2 carb
Wild n Reckless Sherbet	1 scoop	160	2	1	1.5	0	10	40	33	0	1	2 carb

ICE CREAM: REGIONAL FLAVORS

Banana Nut	1 scoop	250	15	5	7	0	45	75	25	1	5	1 1/2 carb, 3 fat
Bananas n Strawberries	1 scoop	230	11	4	7	0	45	85	31	0	4	2 carb, 1 1/2 fat
Black Walnut	1 scoop	280	19	6	9	0	50	90	25	1	6	1 1/2 carb, 3 1/2 fat

✔ = Healthiest Bets

(Continued)

ICE CREAM: REGIONAL FLAVORS *(Continued)*	Amount	Cal.	Fat (g)	% Cal. Fat	Sat. Fat (g)	Trans Fat (g)	Chol. (mg)	Sod. (mg)	Carb. (g)	Fiber (g)	Pro. (g)	Choices/Exchanges
Chocolate Almond	1 scoop	300	18	5	9	0	45	120	32	1	7	2 carb, 3 fat
Chocolate Mousse Royale	1 scoop	310	18	5	13	0	40	140	35	1	5	2 1/2 carb, 3 fat
✓Creole Cream Cheese	1 scoop	190	7	3	4.5	0	25	130	28	0	28	2 carb, 1 1/2 fat
Fudge Brownie	1 scoop	310	18	5	11	0	45	140	35	2	5	2 1/2 carb, 3 fat
Lemon Custard	1 scoop	260	13	5	8	0	75	105	30	0	5	2 carb, 2 1/2 fat
Makin Cookies	1 scoop	310	13	4	9	0	45	180	40	0	4	2 1/2 carb, 2 fat
Mississippi Mud	1 scoop	270	13	4	8	0	45	150	38	1	4	2 1/2 carb, 2 1/2 fat
Oregon Blackberry	1 scoop	250	12	4	8	0	50	85	28	1	4	2 carb, 2 1/2 fat
Rum Raisin	1 scoop	250	11	4	7	0	45	80	34	0	4	2 1/2 carb, 1 1/2 fat
Tiramisu	1 scoop	210	8	3	5	0	35	150	32	0	5	2 carb, 1 fat
ICE CREAM: SEASONAL FLAVORS												
Americas Birthday Cake	1 scoop	280	15	5	10	0	50	105	33	0	4	2 carb, 3 fat

Baseball Nut	1 scoop	280	14	5	8	0	45	160	34	0	5	2 1/2 carb, 3 fat
Cotton Candy	1 scoop	260	12	4	7	0	45	210	32	0	4	2 carb, 2 1/2 fat
Egg Nog	1 scoop	250	13	5	8	0	70	85	31	0	5	2 carb, 2 fat
Everyone's Favorite Candy Bar	1 scoop	250	10	4	5	0	25	190	36	0	5	2 1/2 carb, 2 fat
German Chocolate Cake	1 scoop	300	16	5	9	0	45	150	37	1	5	2 1/2 carb, 2 1/2 fat
Icing on the Cake	1 scoop	290	15	5	10	0.5	45	90	35	0	5	2 1/2 carb, 2 1/2 fat
Love Potion #31	1 scoop	270	14	5	9	0	45	85	32	1	4	2 carb, 2 1/2 fat
✔Peppermint	1 scoop	210	8	3	6	0	25	125	30	0	5	2 carb, 1 fat
Pink Bubblegum	1 scoop	260	12	4	8	0	50	80	36	0	4	2 1/2 carb, 2 fat
✔Pumpkin Pie	1 scoop	180	6	3	4	0	25	125	29	0	4	2 carb, 1/2 fat
Quarterback Crunch	1 scoop	250	12	4	9	0	25	180	33	0	5	2 carb, 2 fat
Strawberry Cheesecake	1 scoop	270	14	5	9	0.5	55	115	32	0	5	2 carb, 3 fat
Tax Crunch	1 scoop	280	15	5	8	0	20	150	32	1	5	2 carb, 2 1/2 fat

✔ = Healthiest Bets

(Continued)

ICE CREAM: SEASONAL FLAVORS *(Continued)*	Amount	Cal.	Fat (g)	% Cal. Fat	Sat. Fat (g)	Trans Fat (g)	Chol. (mg)	Sod. (mg)	Carb. (g)	Fiber (g)	Pro. (g)	Choices/Exchanges
✓Winter White Chocolate	1 scoop	220	9	4	7	0	20	120	30	1	4	2 carb, 2 fat
York Peppermint Pattie	1 scoop	310	18	5	10	0	45	75	37	1	4	2 1/2 carb, 3 fat
SOFT SERVE: 31 BELOW												
Chocolate Oreo	sm (12 oz.)	910	39	4	21	0.5	65	750	131	2	15	8 1/2 carb, 6 fat
Chocolate Oreo	med (16 oz.)	1280	55	4	29	1	85	1060	185	3	21	12 1/2 carb, 9 fat
Chocolate Oreo	lg (24 oz.)	1740	75	4	40	1.5	120	1430	251	4	29	16 1/2 carb, 10 fat
Fudge Brownie	sm (12 oz.)	970	43	4	19	1	125	650	136	1	16	9 carb, 7 fat
Fudge Brownie	med (16 oz.)	1390	62	4	26	1	175	930	194	1	22	13 carb, 10 fat

Fudge Brownie	lg (24 oz.)	1900	85	4	36	1.5	245	1270	265	2	31	17 1/2 carb, 15 fat
Heath	sm (12 oz.)	850	39	4	23	1	85	630	113	1	14	7 1/2 carb, 7 fat
Heath	med (16 oz.)	1150	54	4	31	1	115	840	149	1	19	10 carb, 9 fat
Heath	lg (24 oz.)	1660	77	4	44	1.5	165	1220	219	2	27	14 1/2 carb, 14 fat
Oreo	sm (12 oz.)	710	29	4	15	0.5	65	650	101	2	15	6 1/2 carb, 5 fat
Oreo	med (16 oz.)	980	41	4	21	1	85	900	141	3	20	9 1/2 carb, 7 fat
Oreo	lg (24 oz.)	1350	56	4	29	1.5	120	1230	192	4	28	13 carb, 9 fat
Reese's Peanut Butter Cup	sm (12 oz.)	950	53	5	21	0.5	65	630	97	4	24	6 1/2 carb, 10 fat

✔ = Healthiest Bets

(Continued)

SOFT SERVE: 31 BELOW *(Continued)*

	Amount	Cal.	Fat (g)	% Cal. Fat	Sat. Fat (g)	Trans Fat (g)	Chol. (mg)	Sod. (mg)	Carb. (g)	Fiber (g)	Pro. (g)	Choices/Exchanges
Reese's Peanut Butter Cup	med (16 oz.)	1230	67	5	27	1	90	820	132	5	31	9 carb, 13 fat
Reese's Peanut Butter Cup	lg (24 oz.)	1800	101	5	39	1	125	1190	184	8	45	12 1/2 carb, 19 fat
Strawberry Banana	sm (12 oz.)	530	17	3	11	0.5	65	310	84	3	13	5 1/2 carb, 3 fat
Strawberry Banana	med (16 oz.)	690	23	3	15	0.5	85	420	110	3	18	7 1/2 carb, 3 1/2 fat
Strawberry Banana	lg (24 oz.)	1010	33	3	21	1	120	590	161	5	26	10 1/2 carb, 6 fat
SOFT SERVE: 31 BELOW PIES												
Heath	1 slice	310	14	4	7	0	20	290	43	1	5	3 carb, 2 fat
Oreo	1 slice	290	13	4	6	0	20	290	40	1	5	2 1/2 carb, 2 fat

Reeses Peanut Butter Cup	1 slice	340	18	5	8	0	20	160	38	1	7	2 1/2 carb, 3 fat

SOFT SERVE: CUPS & CONES

Chocolate Dipped Vanilla	kids (3 oz.)	230	14	5	11	0	20	110	24	1	4	1 1/2 carb, 3 fat
Chocolate Dipped Vanilla	reg (6 oz.)	520	33	6	27	0	45	220	51	2	9	3 1/2 carb, 6 fat
Chocolate Dipped Vanilla	lg (9 oz.)	760	47	6	38	0.5	65	330	75	2	13	5 carb, 8 fat
✔ Vanilla	kids (3 oz.)	140	6	4	3.5	0	20	100	19	0	4	1 1/2 carb, 1 fat
Vanilla	reg (6 oz.)	280	11	4	7	0	40	200	37	0	8	2 1/2 carb, 2 fat
Vanilla	lg (9 oz.)	420	17	4	11	0.5	35	300	56	0	12	3 1/2 carb, 3 fat

✔ = Healthiest Bets

(Continued)

	Amount	Cal.	Fat (g)	% Cal. Fat	Sat. Fat (g)	Trans Fat (g)	Chol. (mg)	Sod. (mg)	Carb. (g)	Fiber (g)	Pro. (g)	Choices/Exchanges
SOFT SERVE: FRUIT CREAM												
Berry Pomegranate	sm (12 oz.)	530	15	3	10	0	55	290	89	1	12	6 carb, 2 fat
Berry Pomegranate	med (16 oz.)	670	19	3	12	0.5	70	860	112	1	15	7 1/2 carb, 3 fat
Berry Pomegranate	lg (24 oz.)	920	25	2	16	1	90	470	160	1	19	10 1/2 carb, 4 fat
Mango	sm (12 oz.)	510	14	2	9	0	50	250	89	1	10	6 carb, 2 fat
Mango	med (16 oz.)	640	18	3	11	0.5	65	320	110	1	13	7 1/2 carb, 3 fat
Mango	lg (24 oz.)	890	24	2	15	0.5	85	430	155	2	18	10 1/2 carb, 4 fat

Strawberry Fruit Cream	sm (12 oz.)	530	15	3	10	0	55	290	90	2	12	6 carb, 2 fat
Strawberry Fruit Cream	med (16 oz.)	660	19	3	12	0.5	70	360	112	2	15	7 1/2 carb, 3 fat
Strawberry Fruit Cream	lg (24 oz.)	920	25	2	16	1	90	470	160	3	19	10 1/2 carb, 4 fat

SOFT SERVE: SUNDAES

Caramel	reg (10 oz.)	580	21	3	13	0.5	70	470	89	1	13	6 carb, 3 fat
Caramel	lg (16 oz.)	850	29	3	18	1	100	700	132	1	20	9 carb, 5 fat
Hot Fudge	reg (10 oz.)	620	28	4	17	0	65	400	85	1	13	5 1/2 carb, 5 fat
Hot Fudge	lg (16 oz.)	910	40	4	24	0.5	90	590	126	1	19	8 1/2 carb, 7 fat

(Continued)

✔ = Healthiest Bets

SOFT SERVE: SUNDAES *(Continued)*	Amount	Cal.	Fat (g)	% Cal. Fat	Sat. Fat (g)	Trans Fat (g)	Chol. (mg)	Sod. (mg)	Carb. (g)	Fiber (g)	Pro. (g)	Choices/Exchanges
Strawberry	reg (10 oz.)	450	18	4	11	0	65	310	59	1	12	4 carb, 3 fat
Strawberry	lg (16 oz.)	650	26	4	16	0.5	90	460	87	1	18	6 carb, 4 fat
SUNDAES: CLASSIC SUNDAES												
Banana Royale	1 srvg	630	31	4	18	0.5	85	180	87	3	8	6 carb, 5 fat
Brownie	1 srvg	890	42	4	17	1	150	370	123	1	10	8 carb, 7 fat
Classic Banana Split	1 srvg	980	31	3	18	0.5	100	260	172	8	12	11 1/2 carb, 5 fat
SUNDAES: PREMIUM SUNDAES												
Candy Rush	1 srvg	850	40	4	25	2.5	85	210	115	2	8	7 1/2 carb, 7 fat
Chocolate Oreo	1 srvg	1100	55	5	24	0.5	75	760	151	5	12	10 carb, 10 fat
Heath	1 srvg	1050	50	4	32	1	110	680	142	2	12	9 1/2 carb, 8 fat

Baskin Robbins **113**

Jamoca Oreo	1 srvg	830	32	3	17	1	85	540	130	2	10	8 1/2 carb, 5 fat
Oreo	1 srvg	1330	61	4	31	1	100	950	189	4	14	12 1/2 carb, 10 fat
Reese's Peanut Butter Cup	1 srvg	1250	81	6	32	1	100	680	108	6	27	7 carb, 15 fat
York Peppermint Pattie Brownie	1 srvg	1610	80	4	32	1	195	740	222	3	16	15 carb, 14 fat

✔ = Healthiest Bets

Burger King
(www.burgerking.com)

Light 'n Lean Choice

**Tendergrill Chicken Garden Salad
Ken's Light Italian Dressing *(1 oz, 2 Tbsp)*
Onion Rings *(small)***

Calories	440	Cholesterol (mg)	80
Fat (g)	22	Sodium (mg)	1,150
% calories from fat	45	Carbohydrate (g)	29
Saturated fat (g)	6	Fiber (g)	6
Trans fat (g)	1	Protein (g)	35

Exchanges: 1 starch, 2 veg, 4 lean meat, 2 fat

Healthy 'n Hearty Choice

**Flame Broiled Cheeseburger
French Fries *(small)*
Strawberry Applesauce**

Calories	650	Cholesterol (mg)	55
Fat (g)	29	Sodium (mg)	1,160
% calories from fat	40	Carbohydrate (g)	80
Saturated fat (g)	10	Fiber (g)	3
Trans fat (g)	3.5	Protein (g)	19

Exchanges: 4 starch, 1 fruit, 1 1/2 medium-fat meat, 4 1/2 fat

(Continued)

Burger King

	Amount	Cal.	Fat (g)	% Cal. Fat	Sat. Fat (g)	Trans Fat (g)	Chol. (mg)	Sod. (mg)	Carb. (g)	Fiber (g)	Pro. (g)	Choices/Exchanges
BREAKFAST SANDWICHES												
✔Croissan'wich Bacon, Egg & Cheese	1	340	20	5	7	2	155	890	26	0	15	1 1/2 starch, 1 medium-fat meat, 2 1/2 fat
✔Croissan'wich Egg & Cheese	1	300	17	5	6	2	145	740	26	0	12	1 1/2 starch, 1 medium-fat meat, 2 1/2 fat
Croissan'wich Ham, Egg & Cheese	1	340	18	5	6	2	160	1230	26	1	18	1 1/2 starch, 2 medium-fat meat, 2 fat
Croissan'wich Sausage & Cheese	1	370	25	6	9	2	50	810	23	0	14	1 1/2 starch, 2 high-fat meat, 1 fat
Croissan'wich Sausage, Egg & Cheese	1	470	32	6	11	2.5	180	1060	26	0	19	1 1/2 starch, 3 high-fat meat, 1 fat
Double Croissan'wich Bacon, Egg & Cheese	1	430	27	6	10	2	175	1250	27	0	21	2 starch, 2 medium-fat meat, 3 fat

✔ = Healthiest Bets

(Continued)

BREAKFAST SANDWICHES (*Continued*)	Amount	Cal.	Fat (g)	% Cal. Fat	Sat. Fat (g)	Chol. (mg)	Sod. (mg)	Carb. (g)	Fiber (g)	Pro. (g)	Servings/Exchanges
Double Croissan'wich Ham, Bacon, Egg & Cheese	1	420	24	5	9	2	180	1600	27	1	24	2 starch, 3 medium-fat meat, 2 fat
Double Croissan'wich Ham, Egg & Cheese	1	420	23	5	9	2	185	2210	27	1	27	2 starch, 3 medium-fat meat, 1 1/2 fat
Double Croissan'wich Ham, Sausage, Egg & Cheese	1	550	37	6	15	2.5	205	2040	27	1	28	2 starch, 3 medium-fat meat, 4 fat
Double Croissan'wich Sausage, Bacon, Egg & Cheese	1	550	39	6	14	2.5	200	1420	27	1	25	2 starch, 3 medium-fat meat, 5 fat
Double Croissan'wich Sausage, Egg & Cheese	1	680	51	7	18	3	220	1590	26	1	29	1 1/2 starch, 4 high-fat meat, 3 1/2 fat
Enormous Omelet Sandwich	1	730	45	6	16	1	330	1940	44	2	37	3 starch, 4 medium-fat meat, 5 fat
✔Ham Omelet Sandwich	1	290	13	4	4.5	0	85	870	33	1	13	2 starch, 1 medium-fat meat, 1 1/2 fat

	Amount	Cal.	Fat (g)	% Cal. Fat	Sat. Fat (g)	Trans Fat (g)	Chol. (mg)	Sod. (mg)	Carb. (g)	Fiber (g)	Prot. (g)	Choices/Exchanges
Sausage, Egg & Cheese Biscuit	1	530	37	63	12	6	175	1490	31	1	20	2 starch, 3 high-fat meat, 3 fat
Sausage Biscuit	1	390	26	60	8	5	35	1020	28	1	12	2 starch, 2 high-fat meat, 2 fat

BREAKFAST SIDES

	Amount	Cal.	Fat (g)	% Cal. Fat	Sat. Fat (g)	Trans Fat (g)	Chol. (mg)	Sod. (mg)	Carb. (g)	Fiber (g)	Prot. (g)	Choices/Exchanges
✓ Breakfast Syrup	2 oz	80	0	0	0	0	0	0	20	0	0	1 starch
Cini-minis	1 order	390	18	42	5	4	20	560	51	2	7	3 1/2 starch, 3 fat
French Toast Kid's Meal w/ syrup	1 order	680	24	32	6	3	10	590	100	3	15	6 1/2 starch, 4 fat
French Toast Sticks	3 pc	240	13	49	2.5	2	0	260	26	1	4	1 1/2 starch, 2 1/2 fat
French Toast Sticks	5 pc	390	22	51	4.5	3	0	440	43	2	7	3 starch, 4 fat
✓ Grape Jam	1 oz	30	0	0	0	0	0	0	7	0	0	1/2 starch
Hash Browns	sm	260	17	59	4.5	5	0	500	25	2	2	1 1/2 starch, 3 1/2 fat
Hash Browns	med	430	28	59	8	9	0	830	42	4	4	3 starch, 5 1/2 fat

(Continued)

✓ = Healthiest Bets

BREAKFAST SIDES *(Continued)*	Amount	Cal.	Fat (g)	% Cal. Fat	Sat. Fat (g)	Chol. (mg)	Sod. (mg)	Carb. (g)	Fiber (g)	Pro. (g)	Servings/Exchanges
Hash Browns	lg	620	40	6	11	13	0	1200	60	6	5	4 starch, 8 fat
✓Strawberry Jam	1 oz	30	0	0	0	0	0	0	7	0	0	1/2 starch
Vanilla Icing for Cini-minis	1 order	110	3	2	0.5	0.5	0	40	21	0	0	1 1/2 starch, 1/2 fat
CHICKEN, FISH, AND VEGGIE											
BK Big Fish Sandwich - no tartar sauce	1	470	13	2	3	2	50	1240	65	3	23	4 starch, 2 lean meat, 1 1/2 fat
✓BK Chicken Fries	6 pc	260	15	5	3.5	3	35	650	18	2	12	1 starch, 1 lean meat, 2 1/2 fat
BK Chicken Fries	9 pc	390	23	5	5	1.5	50	980	26	3	18	1 1/2 starch, 2 lean meat, 3 1/2 fat
BK Chicken Fries	12 pc	520	31	5	7	6	65	1300	35	4	25	2 1/2 starch, 3 lean meat, 4 1/2 fat
✓BK Veggie Burger - no mayo	1	340	8	2	1	0	0	1030	46	7	23	3 starch, 2 lean meat, 1/2 fat

BK Veggie Burger w/ cheese	1	470	20	4	5	0	20	1320	47	7	25	3 starch, 2 lean meat, 2 1/2 fat
✔Chicken Tenders	5 pc	210	12	5	3	2	35	600	13	0	12	1 starch, 1 lean meat, 1 1/2 fat
✔Chicken Tenders	8 pc	340	20	5	5	3	55	960	21	0	19	1 1/2 starch, 2 lean meat, 2 1/2 fat
✔Chicken Tenders - Big Kids Meal	6 pc	250	15	5	3.5	2.5	40	720	16	0	14	1 starch, 2 lean meat, 2 fat
✔Chicken Tenders - Kids Meal	4 pc	170	10	5	2.5	1.5	25	180	11	0	9	1/2 starch, 1 lean meat, 1 1/2 fat
Original Chicken Sandwich - no mayo	1	450	17	3	4	2	50	1205	52	4	23	3 1/2 starch, 2 lean meat, 2 1/2 fat
✔Spicy Chick'n Crisp Sandwich - no mayo	1	320	13	4	2.5	1.5	30	730	36	1	15	2 1/2 starch, 1 lean meat, 2 fat
Tendercrisp Chicken Sandwich	1	790	44	5	8	4	70	1640	68	5	33	4 1/2 starch, 3 lean meat, 6 1/2 fat

✔ = Healthiest Bets

(Continued)

CHICKEN, FISH, AND VEGGIE (Continued)	Amount	Cal.	Fat (g)	% Cal. Fat	Sat. Fat (g)	Chol. (mg)	Sod. (mg)	Carb. (g)	Fiber (g)	Pro. (g)	Servings/Exchanges
Tendergrill Chicken Sandwich - no mayo	1	400	7	2	1.5	0	70	1090	49	4	36	3 starch, 3 lean meat
COLD BEVERAGES											
Icee Coca Cola	16 oz	110	0	0	0	0	10	31	0	0	2 carb
Icee Coca Cola	22 oz	140	0	0	0	0	10	40	0	0	2 1/2 carb
Icee Minute Maid Cherry	16 oz	110	0	0	0	0	10	31	0	0	2 carb
Mocha BK Joe Iced Coffee	1	380	10	2	6	0	40	290	66	1	6	4 carb, 2 fat
DESSERTS											
Dutch Apple Pie	1	300	13	4	3	3	0	270	45	1	2	3 carb, 2 1/2 fat
Hershey's Sundae Pie	1	310	19	6	12	0	10	220	32	1	2	2 carb, 4 fat
FLAME BROILED BURGERS											
BK Double Stacker	1	610	39	6	16	1.5	125	1100	32	2	34	2 starch, 4 medium-fat meat, 4 fat

											Servings/Exchanges
BK Quad Stacker	1	1000	68	6	30	3	240	1800	34	1	62	2 1/2 starch, 8 medium-fat meat, 5 1/2 fat
BK Triple Stacker	1	800	54	6	23	2	185	1450	33	1	48	2 starch, 6 medium-fat meat, 5 fat
✔Cheeseburger	1	330	16	4	7	0.5	55	780	31	1	17	2 starch, 2 medium-fat meat, 1 1/2 fat
Double Cheeseburger	1	500	29	5	14	1.5	105	1030	31	1	30	2 starch, 3 medium-fat meat, 2 1/2 fat
Double Hamburger	1	410	21	5	9	1	85	600	30	1	25	2 starch, 3 medium-fat meat, 1 1/2 fat
✔Hamburger	1	290	12	4	4.5	0	40	560	30	1	15	2 starch, 1 medium-fat meat, 1 fat
The Angus Steak Burger	1	640	33	5	10	1.5	185	1260	55	3	33	3 1/2 starch, 3 medium-fat meat, 3 1/2 fat

SALAD DRESSINGS, SAUCES, AND CONDIMENTS

											Servings/Exchanges
Bacon for Whopper Sandwiches	4 strips	50	4	7	1.5	0	10	290	0	0	4	1 fat

(Continued)

✔ = Healthiest Bets

SALAD DRESSINGS, SAUCES, AND CONDIMENTS (*Continued*)	Amount	Cal.	Fat (g)	% Cal. Fat	Sat. Fat (g)	Chol. (mg)	Sod. (mg)	Carb. (g)	Fiber (g)	Pro. (g)	Servings/Exchanges
✓Dipping Sauce - Barbecue	1 oz	40	0	0	0	0	310	11	0	0	1 carb
✓Dipping Sauce - Buffalo	1 oz	80	8	9	1.5	5	350	2	0	0	1 1/2 fat
✓Dipping Sauce - Honey Mustard	1 oz	90	6	6	1	10	180	8	0	0	1/2 carb, 1 fat
Dipping Sauce - Ranch	1 oz	140	15	10	2.5	5	95	1	0	1	3 fat
✓Dipping Sauce - Sweet and Sour	1 oz	45	0	0	0	0	55	11	0	0	1 carb
✓Garlic Parmesan Croutons	1 pkg	60	2	3	0	0	120	9	0	1	1/2 carb, 1/2 fat
Ken's Creamy Caesar Dressing	2 oz	210	21	9	4	25	610	4	0	3	4 fat
✓Ken's Fat Free Ranch Dressing	2 oz	60	0	0	0	0	740	15	2	0	1 carb
Ken's Honey Mustard Dressing	2 oz	270	23	8	3	20	520	15	0	1	1 carb, 4 1/2 fat

	Amount	Cal.	Fat (g)	% Cal. Fat	Sat. Fat (g)	Trans Fat (g)	Chol. (mg)	Sod. (mg)	Carb. (g)	Fiber (g)	Pro. (g)	Servings/Exchanges
✓ Ken's Light Italian Dressing	2 oz	120	11	8	1.5	0	0	440	5	0	0	2 fat
✓ Ken's Ranch Dressing	2 oz	190	20	9	3	0	20	560	2	0	1	4 fat
Zesty Onion Ring Dipping Sauce	1 oz	150	15	9	2.5	0	15	210	3	0	0	3 fat
SALADS												
✓ Garden Salad - no chicken	1	90	5	5	2.5	0	15	125	7	3	5	2 veg
✓ Side Garden Salad	1	15	0	0	0	0	0	0	3	0	1	Free
Tendercrisp Chicken Garden Salad	1	410	22	5	6	3.5	70	1080	26	5	29	1 starch, 2 veg, 4 lean meat, 2 fat
✓ Tendergrill Chicken Garden Salad	1	240	9	3	3	3.5	80	720	8	4	33	2 veg, 4 lean meat
SHAKES												
Chocolate - large	32 oz	950	29	3	19	0.5	115	640	151	2	16	10 carb, 6 fat
Chocolate - medium	22 oz	690	20	3	12	0	75	480	114	2	11	7 1/2 carb, 4 fat

✓ = Healthiest Bets

(Continued)

SHAKES (*Continued*)	Amount	Cal.	Fat (g)	% Cal. Fat	Sat. Fat (g)	Chol. (mg)	Sod. (mg)	Carb. (g)	Fiber (g)	Pro. (g)	Servings/Exchanges
Chocolate - small	16 oz	470	14	3	9	0	55	320	75	1	8	5 carb, 2 1/2 fat
Chocolate - value	12 oz	370	11	3	7	0	42	30	61	1	6	4 carb, 1 1/2 fat
Oreo Sundae Shake Chocolate - medium	22 oz	960	32	3	20	0.5	75	720	154	3	13	10 1/2 carb, 6 1/2 fat
Oreo Sundae Shake Chocolate - small	16 oz	680	24	3	15	0.5	55	480	105	2	9	7 carb, 5 fat
Oreo Sundae Shake Strawberry - medium	22 oz	940	31	3	19	0.5	75	55	151	2	12	10 carb, 6 fat
Oreo Sundae Shake Strawberry - small	16 oz	660	23	3	15	0.5	55	380	103	1	9	7 carb, 4 1/2 fat
Oreo Sundae Shake Vanilla - medium	22 oz	830	33	4	20	1	85	570	119	2	13	8 carb, 6 1/2 fat
Oreo Sundae Shake Vanilla - small	16 oz	610	24	4	16	0.5	60	400	87	1	9	6 carb, 5 fat

Strawberry - large	32 oz	930	28	3	18	0.5	115	490	148	0	15	10 carb, 5 1/2 fat
Strawberry - medium	22 oz	660	19	3	12	0	75	330	111	0	10	7 1/2 carb, 4 fat
Strawberry - small	16 oz	460	14	3	9	0	55	240	73	0	7	5 carb, 3 fat
Strawberry - value	12 oz	360	10	3	7	0	40	180	60	0	6	4 carb, 2 fat
Vanilla - large	32 oz	820	30	3	19	1	125	490	117	0	16	8 carb, 5 1/2 fat
Vanilla - medium	22 oz	560	21	3	13	0.5	85	330	79	0	11	5 1/2 carb, 3 1/2 fat
Vanilla - small	16 oz	400	15	3	9	0	60	240	57	0	8	4 carb, 3 fat
Vanilla - value	12 oz	310	11	3	7	0	45	180	44	0	6	3 carb, 2 fat

SIDE ORDERS

Cheesy Tots Potatoes	6 pc	210	12	5	4.5	2	20	650	20	2	7	1 1/2 starch, 2 1/2 fat
Cheesy Tots Potatoes	9 pc	320	18	5	7	3	30	970	30	2	10	2 starch, 1 high-fat meat, 2 1/2 fat
Cheesy Tots Potatoes	12 pc	430	24	5	9	4	40	1300	40	3	14	2 1/2 starch, 1 high-fat meat, 1 fat

(Continued)

✔ = Healthiest Bets

SIDE ORDERS (*Continued*)	Amount	Cal.	Fat (g)	% Cal. Fat	Sat. Fat (g)	Chol. (mg)	Sod. (mg)	Carb. (g)	Fiber (g)	Pro. (g)	Servings/Exchanges
French Fries, no added salt	sm	230	13	5	3	3	0	240	26	2	2	1 1/2 starch, 2 1/2 fat
French Fries, no added salt	med	360	20	5	4.5	4.5	0	380	41	4	4	2 1/2 starch, 4 fat
French Fries, no added salt	lg	500	28	5	6	6	0	530	57	5	5	4 starch, 5 fat
French Fries, no added salt	king	600	33	5	8	7	0	640	69	6	6	4 1/2 starch, 6 fat
French Fries, salted	sm	230	13	5	3	3	0	380	26	2	2	1 1/2 starch, 2 1/2 fat
French Fries, salted	med	360	20	5	4.5	4.5	0	590	41	4	4	2 1/2 starch, 4 fat
French Fries, salted	lg	500	28	5	6	6	0	820	57	5	5	3 1/2 starch, 5 1/2 fat
French Fries, salted	king	600	33	5	8	7	0	990	69	6	6	4 1/2 starch, 6 fat
✓Mott's Strawberry Flavored Apple Sauce	4 oz	90	0	0	0	0	0	0	23	0	0	1 1/2 carb

Onion Rings	sm	140	7	5	1.5	1	0	210	18	2	2	1 starch, 1 1/2 fat
Onion Rings	med	310	15	4	3.5	2.5	0	440	37	3	4	2 1/2 starch, 3 fat
Onion Rings	lg	440	22	5	4.5	4	0	620	53	5	6	3 1/2 starch, 4 1/2 fat
WHOPPER SANDWICHES												
Double Whopper - no mayo	1	740	39	5	17	2	160	950	51	3	47	3 1/2 starch, 5 medium-fat meat, 2 1/2 fat
Double Whopper w/ cheese - no mayo	1	830	47	5	22	2	180	1380	52	3	52	3 1/2 starch, 6 medium-fat meat, 3 1/2 fat
Triple Whopper - no mayo	1	980	57	5	24	2.5	240	1020	51	3	66	3 1/2 starch, 8 medium-fat meat, 3 1/2 fat
Triple Whopper w/ cheese - no mayo	1	1070	65	5	29	3	260	1450	52	3	71	3 1/2 starch, 9 medium-fat meat, 4 1/2 fat
Whopper - no mayo	1	510	22	4	9	1	80	880	51	3	28	3 1/2 starch, 3 medium-fat meat, 2 fat

(Continued)

✔ = Healthiest Bets

WHOPPER JR. - NO MAYO

	Amount	Cal.	Fat (g)	% Cal. Fat	Sat. Fat (g)	Trans Fat (g)	Chol. (mg)	Sod. (mg)	Carb. (g)	Fiber (g)	Pro. (g)	Choices/Exchanges
✓Whopper Jr. - no mayo	1	290	12	4	4.5	0	40	490	31	2	15	2 starch, 1 medium-fat meat, 1 fat
✓Whopper Jr. w/ cheese - no mayo	1	330	16	4	7	0.5	55	710	31	2	17	2 starch, 2 medium-fat meat, 1 1/2 fat
Whopper w/ cheese - no mayo	1	600	30	5	14	1.5	100	1310	52	3	32	3 1/2 starch, 3 medium-fat meat, 3 fat

✓ = Healthiest Bets

Domino's Pizza
(www.dominos.com)

Light 'n Lean Choice

14" Large Crunchy Thin-Crust Pizza with Green Peppers (*3 slices*)

Calories......................540	Cholesterol (mg).........15
Fat (g) 29	Sodium (mg)..........1,020
% calories from fat..48	Carbohydrate (g).........63
Saturated fat (g) 9	Fiber (g).....................6
Trans fat (g) 0	Protein (g) 21

Exchanges: 4 starch, 1 veg, 2 medium-fat meat, 2 fat

Healthy 'n Hearty Choice

12" Medium Feast, Classic Hand-Tossed Crust Pizza, Vegi Feast (*3 slices*)

Calories......................885	Cholesterol (mg).........25
Fat (g) 42	Sodium (mg)..........2,025
% calories from fat..43	Carbohydrate (g).......102
Saturated fat (g) 18	Fiber (g).....................6
Trans fat (g) 0	Protein (g) 42

Exchanges: 6 starch, 2 veg, 3 medium-fat meat, 5 fat

Domino's Pizza

	Amount	Cal.	Fat (g)	% Cal. Fat	Sat. Fat (g)	Trans Fat (g)	Chol. (mg)	Sod. (mg)	Carb. (g)	Fiber (g)	Pro. (g)	Choices/Exchanges
12" MEDIUM FEAST PIZZAS: OPTIONAL TOPPING												
✓Extra Cheese	1 slice	250	2	1	1	0	4	85	1	0	2	1/2 fat
12" MEDIUM FEAST, CLASSIC HAND-TOSSED CRUST PIZZAS												
America's Favorite Feast	1 slice	345	18	5	7	0	30	785	34	2	15	2 1/2 starch, 1 medium-fat meat, 2 1/2 fat
Bacon Cheeseburger Feast	1 slice	355	19	5	8	0	40	725	33	2	18	2 starch, 2 medium-fat meat, 2 fat
Barbecue Feast	1 slice	345	16	4	7	0	30	695	38	1	16	2 1/2 starch, 1 medium-fat meat, 2 fat
Deluxe Feast	1 slice	315	16	5	6.5	0	25	715	34	2	14	2 1/2 starch, 1 medium-fat meat, 2 fat

ExtravaganZZa	1 slice	375	20	5	8	0	925	35	2	18	2 1/2 starch, 2 medium-fat meat, 2 1/2 fat
Hawaiian Feast	1 slice	305	14	4	6	0	725	35	2	15	2 1/2 starch, 1 medium-fat meat, 1 1/2 fat
MeatZZa Feast	1 slice	365	19	5	8	0	895	34	2	17	2 1/2 starch, 1 medium-fat meat, 2 1/2 fat
Pepperoni Feast	1 slice	345	19	5	8	0	865	34	2	16	2 1/2 starch, 1 medium-fat meat, 2 1/2 fat
Philly Cheese Steak Feast	1 slice	315	15	4	7.5	0	695	31	1	16	2 starch, 1 medium-fat meat, 1 1/2 fat
Vegi Feast	1 slice	295	14	4	6	0	675	34	2	14	2 1/2 starch, 1 medium-fat meat, 2 fat

12" MEDIUM FEAST, CRUNCHY THIN CRUST PIZZAS

America's Favorite Feast	1 slice	265	19	6	6.5	0	690	18	2	11	1 starch, 1 medium-fat meat, 2 1/2 fat

(Continued)

✔ = Healthiest Bets

12" MEDIUM FEAST, CRUNCHY THIN CRUST PIZZAS *(Continued)*	Amount	Cal.	Fat (g)	% Cal. Fat	Sat. Fat (g)	Trans Fat (g)	Chol. (mg)	Sod. (mg)	Carb. (g)	Fiber (g)	Pro. (g)	Choices/Exchanges
Bacon Cheeseburger Feast	1 slice	275	20	7	7.5	0	40	630	17	2	14	1 starch, 2 medium-fat meat, 2 1/2 fat
Barbecue Feast	1 slice	265	17	6	6.5	0	30	600	22	1	12	1 1/2 starch, 1 medium-fat meat, 2 fat
Deluxe Feast	1 slice	235	17	7	6	0	25	620	18	2	10	1 starch, 1 medium-fat meat, 2 1/2 fat
ExtravaganZZa	1 slice	295	21	6	7.5	0	40	830	19	2	14	1 1/2 starch, 1 medium-fat meat, 2 1/2 fat
Hawaiian Feast	1 slice	225	14	6	5.5	0	25	630	19	2	11	1 1/2 starch, 1 medium-fat meat, 2 fat
MeatZZa Feast	1 slice	285	20	6	7.5	0	40	800	18	2	13	1 starch, 1 medium-fat meat, 2 1/2 fat
Pepperoni Feast	1 slice	265	20	7	7.5	0	35	770	18	2	12	1 starch, 1 medium-fat meat, 2 1/2 fat

											Exchanges/Choices
Philly Cheese Steak Feast	1 slice	235	16	6	7	0	30	600	15	1	12	1 starch, 1 medium-fat meat, 2 fat
Vegi Feast	1 slice	215	15	6	5.5	0	25	580	18	2	10	1 starch, 1 medium-fat meat, 2 fat

12" MEDIUM FEAST, ULTIMATE DEEP DISH PIZZAS

America's Favorite Feast	1 slice	360	22	6	7.5	0	30	975	31	4	14	2 starch, 1 medium-fat meat, 3 1/2 fat
Bacon Cheeseburger Feast	1 slice	370	23	6	8.5	0	40	915	30	4	17	2 starch, 2 medium-fat meat, 3 fat
Barbecue Feast	1 slice	360	20	5	7.5	0	30	885	35	3	15	2 1/2 starch, 1 medium-fat meat, 3 fat
Deluxe Feast	1 slice	330	20	5	7	0	25	905	31	4	13	2 starch, 1 medium-fat meat, 3 fat
ExtravaganZZa	1 slice	390	24	6	8.5	0	40	1115	32	4	17	2 starch, 2 medium-fat meat, 3 1/2 fat

(Continued)

✔ = Healthiest Bets

12" MEDIUM FEAST, ULTIMATE DEEP DISH PIZZAS *(Continued)*

	Amount	Cal.	Fat (g)	% Cal. Fat	Sat. Fat (g)	Trans Fat (g)	Chol. (mg)	Sod. (mg)	Carb. (g)	Fiber (g)	Pro. (g)	Choices/Exchanges
Hawaiian Feast	1 slice	320	18	5	6.5	0	25	915	32	4	14	2 starch, 1 medium-fat meat, 2 1/2 fat
MeatZZa Feast	1 slice	380	23	5	8.5	0	40	1085	31	4	16	2 starch, 1 medium-fat meat, 3 fat
Pepperoni Feast	1 slice	360	23	6	8.5	0	35	1055	31	4	15	2 starch, 1 medium-fat meat, 3 1/2 fat
Philly Cheese Steak Feast	1 slice	330	19	5	8	0	30	885	28	3	15	2 starch, 1 medium-fat meat, 2 1/2 fat
Vegi Feast	1 slice	310	18	5	6.5	0	25	865	31	4	13	2 starch, 1 medium-fat meat, 2 1/2 fat

12" MEDIUM, 1 TOPPING, CLASSIC HAND-TOSSED PIZZAS

	Amount	Cal.	Fat (g)	% Cal. Fat	Sat. Fat (g)	Trans Fat (g)	Chol. (mg)	Sod. (mg)	Carb. (g)	Fiber (g)	Pro. (g)	Choices/Exchanges
✔Beef	1 slice	210	9	4	3.5	0	20	420	24	1	9	1 1/2 starch, 1 medium-fat meat, 1 fat
✔Black Olives	1 slice	180	7	4	2	0	10	415	25	1	7	1 1/2 starch, 1 1/2 fat

Food	Serving										Exchanges/Choices
✔Extra Cheese	1 slice	195	8	4	3	0	15	435	25	1	9	1 1/2 starch, 1 medium-fat meat, 1 fat
✔Green Peppers	1 slice	170	6	3	2	0	10	350	24	1	7	1 1/2 starch, 1 fat
✔Ham	1 slice	180	6	3	2	0	15	450	24	1	9	1 1/2 starch, 1 medium-fat meat, 1/2 fat
✔Mushrooms	1 slice	170	6	3	2	0	10	350	24	1	7	1 1/2 starch, 1 fat
✔Onions	1 slice	170	6	3	2	0	10	350	25	1	7	1 1/2 starch, 1 fat
✔Pepperoni	1 slice	210	9	4	3	0	15	490	24	1	9	1 1/2 starch, 1 medium-fat meat, 1 fat
✔Pineapple	1 slice	180	6	3	2	0	10	350	26	1	7	1 1/2 starch, 1 fat
✔Sausage	1 slice	215	9	4	3.5	0	15	480	25	1	9	1 1/2 starch, 1 medium-fat meat, 1 fat

12" MEDIUM, 1 TOPPING, CRUNCHY THIN CRUST PIZZAS

Food	Serving										Exchanges/Choices
Beef	1 slice	170	11	6	4	0	20	310	14	1	7	1 starch, 1 medium-fat meat, 1 1/2 fat

(Continued)

✔ = Healthiest Bets

12" MEDIUM, 1 TOPPING, CRUNCHY THIN CRUST PIZZAS *(Continued)*

	Amount	Cal.	Fat (g)	% Cal. Fat	Sat. Fat (g)	Trans Fat (g)	Chol. (mg)	Sod. (mg)	Carb. (g)	Fiber (g)	Pro. (g)	Choices/Exchanges
✔Black Olives	1 slice	140	9	6	2.5	0	10	305	15	1	5	1 starch, 1 1/2 fat
✔Extra Cheese	1 slice	155	10	6	3.5	0	15	325	15	1	7	1 starch, 1 medium-fat meat, 1 1/2 fat
✔Green Peppers	1 slice	130	8	6	2.5	0	10	240	14	1	5	1 starch, 1 1/2 fat
✔Ham	1 slice	140	8	5	2.5	0	15	340	14	1	7	1 starch, 1 medium-fat meat, 1 fat
✔Mushrooms	1 slice	130	8	6	2.5	0	10	240	14	1	5	1 starch, 1 1/2 fat
✔Onions	1 slice	130	8	6	2.5	0	10	240	15	1	5	1 starch, 1 1/2 fat
Pepperoni	1 slice	170	11	6	3.5	0	15	380	14	1	7	1 starch, 1 medium-fat meat, 1 1/2 fat
✔Pineapple	1 slice	140	8	5	2.5	0	10	240	16	1	5	1 starch, 1 1/2 fat
Sausage	1 slice	175	11	6	4	0	15	370	15	1	7	1 starch, 1 medium-fat meat, 1 1/2 fat

12" MEDIUM, 1 TOPPING, OPTIONAL TOPPINGS

Item	Serving											
American Cheese	1 slice	40	3	7	2	0	10	190	0	0	2	1 fat
✔ Anchovies	1 slice	0	0	0	0	0	0	35	0	0	0	Free
Bacon	1 slice	40	3	7	1	0	10	115	0	0	4	1 medium-fat meat
✔ Banana Peppers	1 slice	0	0	0	0	0	0	130	0	0	0	Free
Cheddar Cheese	1 slice	30	3	9	1.5	0	5	45	0	0	2	1 fat
✔ Chicken Grilled	1 slice	15	0	0	0	0	5	90	0	0	2	Free
✔ Garlic	1 slice	10	0	0	0	0	0	0	1	0	0	Free
✔ Green Chile Peppers	1 slice	0	0	0	0	0	0	0	0	0	0	Free
✔ Green Olive	1 slice	15	2	12	0	0	0	95	0	0	0	Free
✔ Jalapeno	1 slice	0	0	0	0	0	0	100	0	0	0	Free
✔ Philly Meat	1 slice	10	0	0	0	0	5	60	0	0	2	Free
Provolone Cheese	1 slice	45	4	8	0	0	10	110	0	0	3	1 fat

✔ = Healthiest Bets

(Continued)

12" MEDIUM, 1 TOPPING, OPTIONAL TOPPINGS (Continued)

	Amount	Cal.	Fat (g)	% Cal. Fat	Sat. Fat (g)	Trans Fat (g)	Chol. (mg)	Sod. (mg)	Carb. (g)	Fiber (g)	Pro. (g)	Choices/Exchanges
✓Tomatoes	1 slice	5	0	0	0	0		20	1	0	0	Free

12" MEDIUM, 1 TOPPING, ULTIMATE DEEP-DISH PIZZAS

	Amount	Cal.	Fat (g)	% Cal. Fat	Sat. Fat (g)	Trans Fat (g)	Chol. (mg)	Sod. (mg)	Carb. (g)	Fiber (g)	Pro. (g)	Choices/Exchanges
Beef	1 slice	265	14	5	5	0	20	595	27	3	10	2 starch, 1 medium-fat meat, 2 fat
Black Olives	1 slice	235	12	5	3.5	0	10	590	28	3	8	2 starch, 2 1/2 fat
Extra Cheese	1 slice	250	13	5	4.5	0	15	610	28	3	10	2 starch, 1 medium-fat meat, 2 fat
Green Peppers	1 slice	225	11	4	3.5	0	10	525	27	3	8	2 starch, 2 fat
Ham	1 slice	235	11	4	3.5	0	15	625	27	3	10	2 starch, 1 medium-fat meat, 1 1/2 fat
Mushrooms	1 slice	225	11	4	3.5	0	10	525	27	3	8	2 starch, 2 fat
Onions	1 slice	225	11	4	3.5	0	10	525	28	3	8	2 starch, 2 fat
Pepperoni	1 slice	265	15	5	4.5	0	15	665	27	3	10	2 starch, 1 medium-fat meat, 2 fat

	Amount	Cal.	Fat (g)	% Cal. Fat	Sat. Fat (g)	Trans Fat (g)	Chol. (mg)	Sod. (mg)	Carb. (g)	Fiber (g)	Pro. (g)	Servings/Exchanges
Pineapple	1 slice	235	11	42	3.5	0	10	525	29	3	8	2 starch, 2 fat
Sausage	1 slice	270	15	50	5	0	15	655	28	3	10	2 starch, 1 medium-fat meat, 2 1/2 fat
14" BROOKLYN STYLE PIZZA												
Pepperoni	1 slice	330	8	22	4	0.5	35	750	30	2	16	2 starch, 1 medium-fat meat, 2 fat
Sausage	1 slice	350	8	21	4	0.5	35	740	31	2	16	2 starch, 1 medium-fat meat, 2 fat
14" LARGE FEAST PIZZAS: OPTIONAL TOPPING												
Extra Cheese	1 slice	30	2.5	75	1.5	0	5	120	1	0	2	1 fat
14" LARGE FEAST, CLASSIC HAND-TOSSED PIZZAS												
America's Favorite Feast	1 slice	460	23	45	9.5	0	35	1110	48	4	21	3 starch, 2 medium-fat meat, 2 1/2 fat
Bacon Cheeseburger Feast	1 slice	490	24	44	10.5	0	45	1020	46	4	24	3 starch, 2 medium-fat meat, 2 1/2 fat

✓ = Healthiest Bets

(Continued)

14" LARGE FEAST, CLASSIC HAND-TOSSED PIZZAS *(Continued)*

	Amount	Cal.	Fat (g)	% Cal. Fat	Sat. Fat (g)	Trans Fat (g)	Chol. (mg)	Sod. (mg)	Carb. (g)	Fiber (g)	Pro. (g)	Choices/Exchanges
Barbecue Feast	1 slice	460	20	4	8.5	0	35	970	53	3	21	3 1/2 starch, 1 medium-fat meat, 2 fat
Deluxe Feast	1 slice	420	19	4	8.5	0	25	970	47	4	19	3 starch, 1 medium-fat meat, 2 fat
ExtravaganZZa	1 slice	490	25	5	10.5	0	45	1250	49	4	24	3 1/2 starch, 2 medium-fat meat, 3 fat
Hawaiian Feast	1 slice	420	17	4	7.5	0	30	1020	49	4	20	3 1/2 starch, 1 medium-fat meat, 2 fat
MeatZZa Feast	1 slice	500	26	5	11.5	0	45	1280	48	4	24	3 starch, 2 medium-fat meat, 2 1/2 fat
Pepperoni Feast	1 slice	470	24	5	10.5	0	40	1200	47	4	22	3 starch, 2 medium-fat meat, 2 1/2 fat
Philly Cheese Steak Feast	1 slice	420	18	4	9.5	0	35	940	44	3	21	3 starch, 2 medium-fat meat, 2 fat

Vegi Feast	1 slice	410	17	4	7.5	0	25	950	48	4	19	3 starch, 1 medium-fat meat, 2 fat

14" LARGE FEAST, CRUNCHY THIN CRUST PIZZAS

America's Favorite Feast	1 slice	350	24	6	9	0	35	980	26	3	16	1 1/2 starch, 2 medium-fat meat, 2 1/2 fat
Bacon Cheeseburger Feast	1 slice	380	25	6	10	0	45	890	24	3	19	1 1/2 starch, 2 medium-fat meat, 3 fat
Barbecue Feast	1 slice	350	21	5	8	0	35	840	31	2	16	2 starch, 1 medium-fat meat, 2 fat
Deluxe Feast	1 slice	310	20	6	8	0	25	840	25	3	14	1 1/2 starch, 1 medium-fat meat, 2 fat
ExtravaganZZa	1 slice	380	26	6	10	0	45	1120	27	3	19	2 starch, 2 medium-fat meat, 2 1/2 fat
Hawaiian Feast	1 slice	310	18	5	7	0	30	890	27	3	15	2 starch, 1 medium-fat meat, 2 fat

(Continued)

✓ = Healthiest Bets

14" LARGE FEAST, CRUNCHY THIN CRUST PIZZAS *(Continued)*	Amount	Cal.	Fat (g)	% Cal. Fat	Sat. Fat (g)	Trans Fat (g)	Chol. (mg)	Sod. (mg)	Carb. (g)	Fiber (g)	Pro. (g)	Choices/Exchanges
MeatZZa Feast	1 slice	390	27	6	11	0	45	1150	26	3	19	1 1/2 starch, 2 medium-fat meat, 3 fat
Pepperoni Feast	1 slice	360	25	6	10	0	40	1070	25	3	17	1 1/2 starch, 2 medium-fat meat, 2 1/2 fat
Philly Cheese Steak Feast	1 slice	310	19	6	9	0	35	810	22	2	16	1 1/2 starch, 2 medium-fat meat, 2 fat
Vegi Feast	1 slice	300	18	5	7	0	25	820	26	3	14	1 1/2 starch, 1 medium-fat meat, 2 fat
14" LARGE FEAST, ULTIMATE DEEP DISH PIZZAS												
America's Favorite Feast	1 slice	490	28	5	11	0	45	1380	46	6	20	3 starch, 2 medium-fat meat, 3 fat
Bacon Cheeseburger Feast	1 slice	520	29	5	12	0	55	1290	44	6	23	3 starch, 2 medium-fat meat, 3 fat

	Serving									Exchanges
Barbecue Feast	1 slice	490	25	10	0	45	1240	51	5	20	3 1/2 starch, 1 medium-fat meat, 3 fat
Deluxe Feast	1 slice	450	24	10	0	35	1240	45	5	18	3 starch, 1 medium-fat meat, 3 fat
ExtravaganZZa	1 slice	520	30	12	0	55	1520	47	6	23	3 starch, 2 medium-fat meat, 3 fat
Hawaiian Feast	1 slice	450	22	9	0	40	1290	47	6	19	3 starch, 1 medium-fat meat, 3 fat
MeatZZa Feast	1 slice	530	31	13	0	55	1550	46	6	23	3 starch, 2 medium-fat meat, 3 1/2 fat
Pepperoni Feast	1 slice	500	29	12	0	50	1470	45	6	21	3 starch, 2 medium-fat meat, 3 fat
Philly Cheese Steak Feast	1 slice	450	23	11	0	45	1210	42	5	20	3 starch, 2 medium-fat meat, 2 1/2 fat
Vegi Feast	1 slice	440	22	9	0	35	1220	46	6	18	3 starch, 1 medium-fat meat, 3 fat

✔ = Healthiest Bets

(Continued)

14", LARGE, 1 TOPPING, CLASSIC HAND-TOSSED PIZZAS

14" LARGE FEAST, ULTIMATE DEEP DISH PIZZAS (Continued)	Amount	Cal.	Fat (g)	% Cal. Fat	Sat. Fat (g)	Trans Fat (g)	Chol. (mg)	Sod. (mg)	Carb. (g)	Fiber (g)	Pro. (g)	Choices/Exchanges
Beef	1 slice	280	12	4	4.5	0	15	590	34	2	13	2 1/2 starch, 1 medium-fat meat, 1 1/2 fat
Black Olives	1 slice	240	8	3	2.5	0	5	550	35	2	10	2 1/2 starch, 1 1/2 fat
Extra Cheese	1 slice	260	10	3	4	0	10	610	35	2	12	2 1/2 starch, 1 medium-fat meat, 1 1/2 fat
Green Peppers	1 slice	230	8	3	2.5	0	5	490	35	2	10	2 1/2 starch, 1 1/2 fat
Ham	1 slice	245	8	3	2.5	0	10	630	34	2	12	2 1/2 starch, 1 medium-fat meat, 1 fat
Mushrooms	1 slice	230	8	3	2.5	0	5	490	35	2	10	2 1/2 starch, 1 1/2 fat
Onions	1 slice	230	7	3	2.5	0	5	490	35	2	10	2 1/2 starch, 1 1/2 fat
Pepperoni	1 slice	280	12	4	4	0	15	680	34	2	12	2 1/2 starch, 1 medium-fat meat, 1 1/2 fat

Pineapple	1 slice	245	8	3	2.5	0	5	490	37	2	10	2 1/2 starch, 1 1/2 fat
Sausage	1 slice	290	13	4	4.5	0	15	680	36	3	12	2 1/2 starch, 1 medium-fat meat, 2 fat

14" LARGE, 1 TOPPING CRUNCHY THIN CRUST PIZZAS

Beef	1 slice	230	14	5	5	0	15	440	20	2	10	1 1/2 starch, 1 medium-fat meat, 2 fat
✔ Black Olives	1 slice	190	10	5	3	0	5	400	21	2	7	1 1/2 starch, 2 fat
Extra Cheese	1 slice	210	12	5	4.5	0	10	460	21	2	9	1 1/2 starch, 1 medium-fat meat, 1 1/2 fat
✔ Green Peppers	1 slice	180	10	5	3	0	5	340	21	2	7	1 1/2 starch, 2 fat
✔ Ham	1 slice	195	10	5	3	0	10	480	20	2	9	1 1/2 starch, 1 medium-fat meat, 1 1/2 fat
✔ Mushrooms	1 slice	180	10	5	3	0	5	340	21	2	7	1 1/2 starch, 2 fat
Onions	1 slice	180	10	5	3	0	5	340	21	2	7	1 1/2 starch, 2 fat

(Continued)

✔ = Healthiest Bets

14" LARGE, 1 TOPPING, CRUNCHY THIN CRUST PIZZAS (Continued)

	Amount	Cal.	Fat (g)	% Cal. Fat	Sat. Fat (g)	Trans Fat (g)	Chol. (mg)	Sod. (mg)	Carb. (g)	Fiber (g)	Pro. (g)	Choices/Exchanges
Pepperoni	1 slice	230	14	5	4.5	0	15	530	20	2	9	1 1/2 starch, 1 medium-fat meat, 2 fat
✓Pineapple	1 slice	195	10	5	3	0	5	340	23	2	7	1 1/2 starch, 2 fat
Sausage	1 slice	240	15	6	5	0	15	530	22	3	9	1 1/2 starch, 1 medium-fat meat, 2 1/2 fat

14" LARGE, 1 TOPPING, OPTIONAL TOPPINGS

	Amount	Cal.	Fat (g)	% Cal. Fat	Sat. Fat (g)	Trans Fat (g)	Chol. (mg)	Sod. (mg)	Carb. (g)	Fiber (g)	Pro. (g)	Choices/Exchanges
American Cheese	1 slice	45	4	8	2.5	0	10	220	0	0	2	1 fat
✓Anchovies	1 slice	0	0	0	0	0	0	35	0	0	0	Free
Bacon	1 slice	60	4	6	1.5	0	15	170	0	0	6	1 medium-fat meat
✓Banana Peppers	1 slice	0	0	0	0	0	0	180	1	0	0	Free
Cheddar Cheese	1 slice	35	3	8	2	0	10	55	0	0	2	1 fat
✓Chicken Grilled	1 slice	20	1	5	0	0	10	130	0	0	3	1/2 fat
✓Garlic	1 slice	15	0	0	0	0	0	0	1	0	0	Free

Item	Amount	Cal.	Fat (g)	% Cal. Fat	Sat. Fat (g)	Trans Fat (g)	Chol. (mg)	Sod. (mg)	Carb. (g)	Fiber (g)	Pro. (g)	Servings/Exchanges
✔ Green Chile Peppers	1 slice	0	0	0	0		0	0	0	0	0	Free
✔ Green Olive	1 slice	20	2	9	0		0	125	1	0	0	1/2 fat
✔ Jalapeno	1 slice	0	0	0	0		0	135	0	0	0	Free
✔ Philly Meat	1 slice	15	1	6	0		5	85	0	0	2	Free
✔ Provolone Cheese	1 slice	60	5	8	3		10	160	0	0	5	1 medium-fat meat
✔ Tomatoes	1 slice	0	0	0	0		0	25	1	0	0	Free
14" LARGE, 1 TOPPING, ULTIMATE DEEP DISH PIZZAS												
Beef	1 slice	370	19	5	7	0	25	840	40	5	14	2 1/2 starch, 1 medium-fat meat, 3 fat
Black Olives	1 slice	330	15	4	5	0	15	800	41	5	11	2 1/2 starch, 3 fat
Extra Cheese	1 slice	350	17	4	6.5	0	20	860	41	5	13	2 1/2 starch, 1 medium-fat meat, 2 1/2 fat
Green Peppers	1 slice	320	14	4	5	0	15	740	41	5	11	2 1/2 starch, 3 fat

(Continued)

✔ = Healthiest Bets

14" LARGE, 1 TOPPING, ULTIMATE DEEP DISH PIZZAS *(Continued)*

	Amount	Cal.	Fat (g)	% Cal. Fat	Sat. Fat (g)	Trans Fat (g)	Chol. (mg)	Sod. (mg)	Carb. (g)	Fiber (g)	Pro. (g)	Choices/Exchanges
Ham	1 slice	335	15	4	5	0	20	880	40	5	13	2 1/2 starch, 1 medium-fat meat, 2 fat
Mushrooms	1 slice	320	14	4	5	0	15	740	41	5	11	2 1/2 starch, 3 fat
Onions	1 slice	320	14	4	5	0	15	740	41	5	11	2 1/2 starch, 3 fat
Pepperoni	1 slice	370	19	5	6.5	0	25	930	40	5	13	2 1/2 starch, 1 medium-fat meat, 3 fat
Pineapple	1 slice	335	14	4	5	0	15	740	43	5	11	3 starch, 3 fat
Sausage	1 slice	380	20	5	7	0	25	930	42	6	13	3 starch, 1 medium-fat meat, 3 fat
16" BROOKLYN STYLE PIZZA												
Pepperoni	1 slice	460	11	2	5	1	45	990	43	3	22	3 starch, 2 medium-fat meat, 2 fat
Sausage	1 slice	480	11	2	6	0.5	45	1000	44	3	22	3 starch, 2 medium-fat meat, 2 1/2 fat

SIDE ITEMS: BREAD

Item	Amount	Cal.	Fat (g)	% Cal. Fat	Sat. Fat (g)	Trans Fat (g)	Chol. (mg)	Sod. (mg)	Carb. (g)	Fiber (g)	Prot. (g)	Servings/Exchanges
Breadsticks	1 stick	110	6	5	1.5	0	0	100	11	0	2	1/2 starch, 1 fat
Cheesy Bread	1 stick	120	6	5	2	0	5	150	11	0	4	1/2 starch, 1 fat
Cinna Stix	1 stick	120	6	5	1	0	0	85	14	1	2	1 starch, 1 fat

SIDE ITEMS: BREAD DIPPING SAUCES

Item	Amount	Cal.	Fat (g)	% Cal. Fat	Sat. Fat (g)	Trans Fat (g)	Chol. (mg)	Sod. (mg)	Carb. (g)	Fiber (g)	Prot. (g)	Servings/Exchanges
Garlic Dipping Sauce	2 oz.	440	49	10	10	7	0	390	0	0	0	10 fat
✓ Marinara Dipping Sauce	2 oz.	25	0	0	0	0	0	260	5	1	1	1/2 carb
Sweet Icing Dipper Cup	2.5 oz.	250	3	1	2.5	0	0	0	57	0	0	4 carb

SIDE ITEMS: CHICKEN

Item	Amount	Cal.	Fat (g)	% Cal. Fat	Sat. Fat (g)	Trans Fat (g)	Chol. (mg)	Sod. (mg)	Carb. (g)	Fiber (g)	Prot. (g)	Servings/Exchanges
Barbeque Buffalo Wings	2 pieces	230	14	5	3.5	0	50	410	6	0	17	1/2 starch, 2 lean meat, 1 1/2 fat
✓ Buffalo Chicken Kickers	2 pieces	90	3	3	0.5	0	20	90	6	1	9	1/2 starch, 1 lean meat
Hot Buffalo Wings	2 pieces	210	14	6	3.5	0	50	440	5	0	16	1/2 starch, 2 lean meat, 1 1/2 fat

✓ = Healthiest Bets

(Continued)

	Amount	Cal.	Fat (g)	% Cal. Fat	Sat. Fat (g)	Chol. (mg)	Sod. (mg)	Carb. (g)	Fiber (g)	Pro. (g)	Servings/Exchanges
SIDE ITEMS: CHICKEN DIPPING SAUCES											
Blue Cheese Dipping Cup	1.5 oz.	210	22	9	4	0	20	390	2	0	1	4 1/2 fat
Hot Dipping Cup	1.5 oz.	120	12	9	2	0	0	790	3	0	0	3 fat
Ranch Dipping Cup	1.5 oz.	190	21	10	3	0	10	390	2	0	1	4 fat
SIDE ITEMS: SALAD DRESSINGS											
Blue Cheese Dressing	1.5 oz.	230	24	9	5	0	30	450	2	0	2	5 fat
Buttermilk Ranch Dressing	1.5 oz.	220	24	10	4	0	10	420	2	0	1	5 fat
Creamy Caesar Dressing	1.5 oz.	210	22	9	3.5	0	10	510	2	0	1	4 1/2 fat
✔Golden Italian Dressing	1.5 oz.	220	23	9	3.5	0	0	370	2	0	0	4 1/2 fat
✔Light Italian Dressing	1.5 oz.	20	1	5	0	0	0	780	2	0	0	Free

SIDE ITEMS: SALADS

	Amount											Exchanges
✔ Garden Fresh Salad	1 salad	70	4	5	2.5	0	10	80	5	2	4	1 veg, 1 fat
✔ Grilled Chicken Caesar Salad	1 salad	100	5	5	2	0	20	310	6	2	10	1 veg, 1 lean meat

✔ = Healthiest Bets

Dunkin' Donuts
(www.dunkindonuts.com)

Light 'n Lean Choice

Egg Cheese English Muffin
Orange Juice

Calories	365	Cholesterol (mg)	190
Fat (g)	13	Sodium (mg)	1,081
% calories from fat	32	Carbohydrate (g)	47
Saturated fat (g)	5	Fiber (g)	0
Trans fat (g)	0	Protein (g)	15

Exchanges: 2 starch, 1 high-fat meat, 1 fruit, 1 fat

Healthy 'n Hearty Choice

Glazed Cake Donuts *(2)*
Latte *(10 oz)*

Calories	580	Cholesterol (mg)	25
Fat (g)	26	Sodium (mg)	735
% calories from fat	40	Carbohydrate (g)	70
Saturated fat (g)	14	Fiber (g)	2
Trans fat (g)	0	Protein (g)	14

Exchanges: 4 carb, 1 milk, 1/2 fat

Dunkin' Donuts

	Amount	Cal.	Fat (g)	% Cal. Fat	Sat. Fat (g)	Trans Fat (g)	Chol. (mg)	Sod. (mg)	Carb. (g)	Fiber (g)	Pro. (g)	Choices/Exchanges
BAGELS												
Blueberry	1	330	3	1	1	0	0	600	66	2	10	4 1/2 starch, 1/2 fat
Cinnamon Raisin	1	330	3	1	1	0	0	430	65	3	10	4 starch, 1/2 fat
Everything	1	370	6	1	1	0	0	650	67	3	14	4 1/2 starch, 1 fat
Multigrain	1	380	6	1	1	0	0	650	68	5	14	4 1/2 starch, 1 fat
Onion	1	320	4	1	1	0	0	610	61	3	12	4 starch, 1/2 fat
Plain	1	320	3	1	1	0	0	650	62	2	12	4 starch, 1/2 fat
Poppy seed	1	370	7	2	1	0	0	650	65	3	14	4 starch, 1 fat
Salt	1	320	3	1	1	0	0	4520	62	2	12	4 starch, 1/2 fat
Sesame	1	380	8	2	1	0	0	650	64	3	14	4 starch, 1 fat

(Continued)

✔ = Healthiest Bets

BAGELS *(Continued)*	Amount	Cal.	Fat (g)	% Cal. Fat	Sat. Fat (g)	Trans Fat (g)	Chol. (mg)	Sod. (mg)	Carb. (g)	Fiber (g)	Pro. (g)	Choices/Exchanges
Wheat	1	330	4	1	1	0	0	610	62	4	12	4 starch, 1/2 fat
BREAKFAST SANDWICHES												
Bacon Egg Cheese Bagel	1	540	18	3	7	0	200	1400	69	2	18	4 1/2 starch, 1 medium-fat meat, 2 1/2 fat
Bacon Egg Cheese Croissant	1	440	25	5	12	0	150	910	33	1	19	2 starch, 2 high-fat meat, 2 fat
Bacon Egg Cheese English Muffin	1	360	16	4	6	0	200	1300	36	0	17	2 starch, 2 high-fat meat
Bacon Lover's Supreme	1	640	43	6	19	1	280	1120	36	2	26	2 starch, 3 high-fat meat, 4 fat
Egg Cheese Bagel	1	470	15	3	6	0	190	1120	65	2	20	4 starch, 1 high-fat meat, 1 1/2 fat
Egg Cheese Biscuit	1	540	29	5	17	0	125	1390	53	2	16	3 1/2 starch, 1 high-fat meat, 4 fat

Egg Cheese Croissant	1	430	26	5	11	0	190	780	33	1	14	2 starch, 1 high-fat meat
Egg Cheese English Muffin	1	310	13	4	5	0	190	1080	35	1	14	2 starch, 1 high-fat meat, 1 fat
Ham Egg Cheese Bagel	1	510	16	3	6	0	200	1390	65	2	26	4 starch, 2 medium-fat meat, 1 fat
Ham Egg Cheese Croissant	1	460	27	5	12	0	205	1040	33	1	20	2 starch, 2 medium-fat meat, 3 1/2 fat
Ham Egg Cheese English Muffin	1	310	10	3	5	0	160	1270	34	1	21	2 starch, 2 medium-fat meat
Hash Browns	9 pcs	180	9	5	1	0	0	730	22	3	2	1 1/2 starch, 2 fat
Sausage Egg Cheese Bagel	1	660	35	5	13	.5	225	1450	63	3	28	4 starch, 2 high-fat meat, 3 1/2 fat
Sausage Egg Cheese Biscuit	1	800	32	4	24	0	235	1960	54	2	24	3 1/2 starch, 2 high-fat meat, 3 fat
Sausage Egg Cheese Croissant	1	630	45	6	17	1	230	1250	34	1	24	2 starch, 2 high-fat meat, 6 fat

✔ = Healthiest Bets

(Continued)

BREAKFAST SANDWICHES *(Continued)*	Amount	Cal.	Fat (g)	% Cal. Fat	Sat. Fat (g)	Trans Fat (g)	Chol. (mg)	Sod. (mg)	Carb. (g)	Fiber (g)	Pro. (g)	Choices/Exchanges
Sausage Egg Cheese English Muffin	1	530	32	5	12	.5	235	1610	37	1	23	2 1/2 starch, 3 high-fat meat, 1 fat
Supreme Omelet Sandwich on a Croissant	1	530	33	6	14	0	255	1070	35	2	21	2 starch, 2 medium-fat meat, 5 fat
COOKIES												
Chocolate Chunk	4.5 oz	540	23	4	13	0	50	550	80	3	7	5 carb, 4 1/2 fat
Oatmeal Raisin Pecan	4.5 oz	480	14	3	7	0	40	310	83	5	8	5 carb, 3 fat
Peanut Butter Cup	4.5 oz	590	29	4	13	0	50	530	73	3	11	5 carb, 6 fat
COOLATTA												
Cherry Lime SoBe	16 oz	250	0	0	0	0	0	65	62	2	0	4 carb
Coffee w/ 2% milk	16 oz	190	2	1	1.5	0	10	80	41	0	4	2 1/2 carb
Coffee w/ cream	16 oz	350	22	6	14	0	75	65	40	0	3	2 1/2 carb, 4 fat

	Amount	Cal	Fat (g)	% Cal Fat	Sat Fat (g)	Trans Fat (g)	Chol (mg)	Sod (mg)	Carb (g)	Fiber (g)	Pro (g)	Exchanges/Choices
Coffee w/ milk	16 oz	210	4	2	2.5	0	15	80	42	0	4	3 carb, 1 fat
Coffee w/ skim milk	16 oz	170	0	0	0	0	0	80	41	0	4	3 carb
Lemonade	16 oz	240	0	0	0	0	0	35	59	0	0	4 carb
Strawberry Fruit	16 oz	290	0	0	0	0	0	30	72	1	0	4 1/2 carb
Tropicana Orange	16 oz	370	0	0	0	0	0	50	92	3	1	6 carb
Vanilla Bean	16 oz	500	17	3	17	0	0	95	85	2	1	5 carb, 3 fat

CRAVINGS SANDWICHES

	Amount	Cal	Fat (g)	% Cal Fat	Sat Fat (g)	Trans Fat (g)	Chol (mg)	Sod (mg)	Carb (g)	Fiber (g)	Pro (g)	Exchanges/Choices
Chicken Bruschetta	1	580	25	4	8	0	85	1450	48	4	42	3 starch, 5 lean meat, 2 fat
Chipotle Chicken	1	620	26	4	9	0	110	1730	49	4	49	3 starch, 6 lean meat, 1 1/2 fat
Pastrami Supreme	1	760	42	5	17	0	130	1990	47	5	48	3 starch, 6 medium-fat meat, 2 1/2 fat
Turkey Pesto	1	530	23	4	8	0	65	1630	48	4	33	3 starch, 3 lean meat, 3 fat

✓ = Healthiest Bets

(Continued)

	Amount	Cal.	Fat (g)	% Cal. Fat	Sat. Fat (g)	Trans Fat (g)	Chol. (mg)	Sod. (mg)	Carb. (g)	Fiber (g)	Pro. (g)	Choices/Exchanges
CREAM CHEESE												
✓Chive	4 T	170	17	9	11	0	45	230	4	2	4	3 fat
✓Garden Vegetable	4 T	170	15	8	11	0	45	340	4	0	2	3 1/2 fat
✓Lite	4 T	120	9	7	6	0	30	280	5	0	4	2 fat
✓Lite Garden Vegetable	4 T	100	8	7	5	0	25	270	5	0	3	1 1/2 fat
✓Plain	4 T	190	17	8	13	0	55	190	4	0	4	3 1/2 fat
Reduced Carb w/ Cheese	1	380	12	3	5	0	20	780	45	14	25	3 starch, 2 1/2 fat
✓Salmon	4 T	170	17	9	11	0	45	180	2	0	4	3 1/2 fat
✓Strawberry	4 T	190	17	8	9	0	45	150	9	0	4	3 1/2 fat
DANISH												
Apple	1	330	20	5	9	0	30	260	32	1	4	2 carb, 4 fat
Cheese	1	340	22	6	10	0	35	270	30	1	4	2 carb, 4 1/2 fat

Item												Servings/Exchanges
Strawberry Cheese	1	320	20	6	9	0	30	260	31	1	4	2 carb, 4 fat

DELI CLASSICS SANDWICHES

Item												Servings/Exchanges
Ham and Swiss	1	360	11	3	5	0	45	1120	44	4	23	3 starch, 2 lean meat, 1 fat
Roast Beef and Swiss	1	530	25	4	8	0	80	1290	45	4	31	3 starch, 3 lean meat, 3 fat
Tuna	1	550	26	4	5	0	35	830	49	4	29	3 starch, 3 lean meat, 3 fat
Turkey and Cheese	1	510	22	4	6	0	65	1380	45	4	35	3 starch, 4 lean meat, 2 fat
Vegetarian	1	420	21	5	3	0	5	480	51	8	9	3 starch, 1 veg, 4 fat

DONUTS

Item												Servings/Exchanges
✓ Gingerbread	1	280	4	1	1	0	45	400	56	1	5	3 1/2 carb, 1 fat
Wheat Glazed Cake	1	310	19	6	8	0	0	380	32	2	4	2 carb, 4 fat
Apple Crumb	1	320	13	4	6	0	0	360	45	2	4	3 carb, 2 1/2 fat
Apple N' Spice	1	260	11	4	5	0	0	350	35	2	4	2 carb, 2 fat
Bavarian Kreme	1	250	6	2	6	0	20	460	52	1	4	3 1/2 carb, 1 fat

✓ = Healthiest Bets

(*Continued*)

DONUTS *(Continued)*	Amount	Cal.	Fat (g)	% Cal. Fat	Sat. Fat (g)	Trans Fat (g)	Chol. (mg)	Sod. (mg)	Carb. (g)	Fiber (g)	Pro. (g)	Choices/Exchanges
✔Black Raspberry	1	270	10	3	5	0	0	350	40	1	4	2 1/2 carb, 2 fat
Blueberry Cake	1	290	16	5	6	0	10	400	35	1	3	2 carb, 3 fat
Blueberry Crumb	1	330	13	4	6	0	0	360	48	2	4	3 carb, 2 1/2 fat
Boston Kreme	1	270	12	4	5	0	0	370	38	1	4	2 1/2 carb, 3 fat
Chocolate Coconut	1	370	21	5	11	0	0	380	42	3	3	3 carb, 4 fat
Chocolate Frosted	1	330	19	5	9	0	15	260	36	2	4	2 1/2 carb, 4 fat
Chocolate Glazed	1	340	19	5	9	0	0	360	39	2	3	2 1/2 carb, 4 fat
Chocolate Kreme Filled	1	300	14	4	6	0	0	360	39	2	4	2 1/2 carb, 3 fat
Cinnamon	1	310	18	5	9	0	15	260	34	2	3	2 carb, 3 1/2 fat
Double Chocolate	1	340	20	5	9	0	0	360	36	3	3	2 carb, 4 fat
✔French Cruller	1	150	8	5	5	0	20	105	17	1	2	1 carb, 2 1/2 fat
Glazed	1	330	18	5	9	0	15	260	38	2	3	2 1/2 carb, 3 1/2 fat
✔Glazed Cake	1	230	10	4	5	0	0	320	30	1	4	2 carb

✔ Jelly Filled	1	270	10	3	5	0	0	350	39	1	4	2 1/2 carb, 2 fat
✔ Maple Frosted	1	240	10	4	5	0	0	320	31	1	4	2 carb, 2 fat
Marble Frosted	1	230	11	4	5	0	0	320	30	1	4	2 carb, 2 fat
Mini M&M	1	270	12	4	5	0	0	360	39	1	4	2 1/2 carb, 2 1/2 fat
Old Fashioned Cake	1	280	18	6	9	0	15	260	26	2	3	1 1/2 carb, 3 1/2 fat
Powdered	1	310	18	5	9	0	15	260	34	2	3	3 carb, 3 1/2 fat
Pumpkin Glazed	1	280	6	2	6	0	20	460	52	1	4	3 1/2 carb, 1 fat
✔ Strawberry Frosted	1	240	10	4	5	0	0	330	32	1	4	2 carb, 2 fat
✔ Sugar Raised	1	210	10	4	5	0	0	320	27	1	4	2 carb, 2 fat
Vanilla Kreme Filled	1	320	16	5	7	0	0	360	39	1	4	2 1/2 carb, 3 fat
FANCIES												
Apple Fritter	1	290	13	4	6	0	0	360	35	2	4	2 carb, 2 1/2 fat
Bow Tie Donut	1	300	17	5	8	0	0	340	34	1	4	2 carb, 3 fat

✔ = Healthiest Bets

(Continued)

FANCIES *(Continued)*	Amount	Cal.	Fat (g)	% Cal. Fat	Sat. Fat (g)	Trans Fat (g)	Chol. (mg)	Sod. (mg)	Carb. (g)	Fiber (g)	Pro. (g)	Choices/Exchanges
Chocolate Frosted Coffee Roll	1	340	20	5	9	0	0	340	36	1	4	2 carb, 4 fat
Chocolate Iced Bismarck	1	340	15	4	6	0	0	290	50	1	3	3 1/2 carb, 3 fat
Coffee Roll	1	340	20	5	9	0	0	340	33	1	4	2 carb, 4 fat
Éclair	1	300	15	5	6	0	0	260	39	1	3	2 1/2 carb, 3 fat
Glazed Fritter	1	250	13	5	6	0	0	330	31	1	4	2 carb, 2 1/2 fat
Maple Frosted Coffee Roll	1	340	20	5	9	0	0	340	36	1	4	2 carb, 4 fat
Vanilla Frosted Coffee Roll	1	340	20	5	9	0	0	340	36	1	4	2 carb, 4 fat
FAVORITES SANDWICHES												
Avocado and Turkey	1	500	22	4	3	0	40	1330	49	8	38	3 starch, 4 lean meat, 2 fat
Chicken Cordon Bleu	1	550	19	3	7	0	95	1370	51	4	45	3 starch, 5 lean meat, 1 fat
Steak and Cheese	1	510	23	4	6	0	75	1830	45	4	30	3 starch, 3 medium-fat meat, 1 1/2 fat

	Amount	Cal.	Fat (g)	Sat. Fat (g)	% Fat Cal.	Trans Fat (g)	Chol. (mg)	Sod. (mg)	Carb. (g)	Fiber (g)	Pro. (g)	Choices/Exchanges
Toasted Italian	1	630	34	5	12	0	90	2330	49	5	35	3 starch, 5 medium-fat meat, 2 fat

FLAT BREAD SANDWICHES

	Amount	Cal.	Fat (g)	Sat. Fat (g)	% Fat Cal.	Trans Fat (g)	Chol. (mg)	Sod. (mg)	Carb. (g)	Fiber (g)	Pro. (g)	Choices/Exchanges
Ham and Swiss	1	350	12	3	5	0	35	1040	41	2	20	3 starch, 2 lean meat, 1 fat
Three Cheese	1	460	24	5	12	0	55	1000	42	2	20	3 starch, 2 high-fat meat, 1/2 fat
Turkey, Cheddar and Bacon	1	360	13	3	5	0	35	1060	41	2	20	3 starch, 2 lean meat, 1 fat

HOT CHOCOLATE

	Amount	Cal.	Fat (g)	Sat. Fat (g)	% Fat Cal.	Trans Fat (g)	Chol. (mg)	Sod. (mg)	Carb. (g)	Fiber (g)	Pro. (g)	Choices/Exchanges
Dunkaccino	10 oz	230	11	4	9	0	10	5	35	0	2	2 carb, 2 fat
Hot Chocolate	10 oz	230	7	3	7	0	0	290	39	2	2	2 1/2 carb, 2 fat
Milky Way Hot Chocolate	10 oz	200	7	3	6	0	0	410	37	1	1	2 1/2 carb
Vanilla Chai	10 oz	230	8	3	6	0	5	50	40	0	1	3 carb
White Hot Chocolate	10 oz	230	9	4	7	0	0	290	37	0	2	2 1/2 carb

(Continued)

✔ = Healthiest Bets

HOT ESPRESSO DRINKS

	Amount	Cal.	Fat (g)	% Cal. Fat	Sat. Fat (g)	Trans Fat (g)	Chol. (mg)	Sod. (mg)	Carb. (g)	Fiber (g)	Pro. (g)	Choices/Exchanges
✔Cappuccino	10 oz	80	5	6	2.5	0	20	70	7	0	4	1 milk
✔Cappuccino w/ Soy Milk	10 oz	70	3	4	0	0	0	80	6	1	4	1 milk
✔Cappuccino w/ Soy Milk & Sugar	10 oz	120	3	2	0	0	0	80	20	1	4	1/2 carb, 1 milk
✔Cappuccino w/ Sugar	10 oz	130	5	3	2.5	0	15	65	21	0	4	1/2 carb, 1 milk, 1 fat
Caramel Cream Latte	10 oz	260	9	3	6	0	20	125	40	0	8	2 carb, 1 milk, 2 fat
Caramel Swirl Latte	10 oz	230	6	2	3.5	0	25	140	36	0	8	2 carb, 1 milk
Caramel Swirl Latte w/ Soy Milk	10 oz	210	4	2	0	0	0	160	34	1	8	1 1/2 carb, 1 milk
✔Espresso	2 oz	0	0	0	0	0	0	5	1	0	0	Free
✔Espresso w/ Sugar	2 oz	30	0	0	0	0	0	5	7	0	0	1/2 carb
Gingerbread Latte	10 oz	330	9	2	5	0	30	160	54	0	9	3 carb, 1 milk, 2 fat

✔Hot Latte Lite	10 oz	70	0	0	0	50	80	10	0	6	1 milk
✔Latte	10 oz	120	6	3.5	0	25	95	10	0	6	1 milk, 1/2 fat
✔Latte w/ Soy Milk	10 oz	90	4	0	0	0	110	8	1	6	1 milk
✔Latte w/ Soy Milk & Sugar	10 oz	150	4	0	0	0	110	22	1	6	1/2 carb, 1 milk
Latte w/ Sugar	10 oz	160	6	3.5	0	25	95	22	0	6	1/2 carb, 1 milk, 1 fat
Mocha Almond Latte	10 oz	290	10	7	0	20	115	46	1	8	2 carb, 1 milk, 2 fat
Mocha Swirl Latte	10 oz	230	7	4	0	25	110	37	1	6	2 carb, 1/2 milk, 1 fat
Mocha Swirl Latte w/ Soy Milk	10 oz	210	5	2	1	0	130	35	2	7	2 carb, 1/2 milk, 1 fat
Pumpkin Spice Latte	10 oz	220	6	2	3.5	20	130	34	0	8	1 1/2 carb, 1 milk
Turbo Hot Latte	10 oz	130	6	4	3.5	20	55	20	0	1	1/2 carb, 1 milk
✔Vanilla Latte Lite	10 oz	80	0	0	0	5	80	10	0	6	1 milk

✔ = Healthiest Bets

(Continued)

ICED ESPRESSO DRINKS

	Amount	Cal.	Fat (g)	% Cal. Fat	Sat. Fat (g)	Trans Fat (g)	Chol. (mg)	Sod. (mg)	Carb. (g)	Fiber (g)	Pro. (g)	Choices/Exchanges
Iced Caramel Cream Latte	16 oz	260	9	3	6	0	20	125	40	0	8	2 carb, 1 milk
Iced Caramel Swirl Latte	16 oz	240	7	3	4	0	25	150	37	0	8	1 1/2 carb, 1 milk, 1 fat
Iced Caramel Swirl Latte w/ fat-free milk	16 oz	180	0	0	0	0	0	150	36	0	8	1 1/2 carb, 1 milk
✓Iced Latte	16 oz	120	7	5	4	0	25	105	11	0	6	1 milk
✓Iced Latte Lite	16 oz	80	0	0	0	0	0	110	13	0	7	1 milk
✓Iced Latte w/ fat-free milk	16 oz	70	0	0	0	0	0	110	11	0	7	1 milk
✓Iced Latte w/ fat-free milk and sugar	16 oz	120	0	0	0	0	0	110	23	0	7	1/2 carb, 1 milk
✓Iced Latte w/ Sugar	16 oz	170	7	4	4	0	25	110	23	0	6	1 carb, 1 milk
Iced Mocha Almond Latte	16 oz	290	10	3	7	0	20	115	46	1	8	2 carb, 1 milk

Iced Mocha Swirl Latte	16 oz	240	8	3	4.5	0	25	125	38	1	7	1 1/2 carb, 1 milk
Iced Mocha Swirl Latte w/ fat-free milk	16 oz	180	1	1	1	0	0	115	37	1	7	1 1/2 carb, 1 milk
Turbo Ice	16 oz	120	7	5	3.5	0	20	25	14	0	1	1 carb, 1 1/2 fat

MUFFINS & MISC.

Banana Walnut Muffin	1	540	25	4	3.5	0	65	520	69	3	10	4 1/2 carb, 4 fat
Biscuit	1	440	22	5	13	0	0	980	51	2	7	3 1/2 starch, 4 1/2 fat
Blueberry Muffin	1	470	17	3	3	0	60	500	73	2	8	5 carb, 2 fat
Chocolate Chip Muffin	1	630	26	4	8	0	70	560	89	2	10	5 1/2 carb, 4 fat
Cinnamon Cake	4	270	15	5	3.5	4	25	210	31	1	3	2 carb, 2 1/2 fat
Coffee Cake Muffin	1	580	19	3	3	0	65	520	78	1	9	5 carb, 4 fat
Corn Muffin	1	510	18	3	3.5	0	75	860	77	1	8	5 carb, 3 fat
Cranberry Orange Muffin	1	440	17	3	3	0	65	480	66	3	8	4 1/2 carb, 3 fat

(Continued)

✔ = Healthiest Bets

MUFFINS & MISC. *(Continued)*	Amount	Cal.	Fat (g)	% Cal. Fat	Sat. Fat (g)	Trans Fat (g)	Chol. (mg)	Sod. (mg)	Carb. (g)	Fiber (g)	Pro. (g)	Choices/Exchanges
Croissant	1	27	14	47	6	0	0	300	30	1	6	2 starch, 3 fat
✔English Muffin	1	160	1.5	1	0	0	0	340	31	2	1	2 starch
Honey Bran Raisin Muffin	1	480	15	3	2.5	0	60	480	79	5	8	5 carb, 2 fat
Reduced Fat Blueberry Muffin	1	400	5	1	2	0	60	480	78	3	8	5 carb, 1 fat
MUNCHKINS												
Cinnamon Cake	4	260	15	5	7	0	10	210	29	2	3	2 carb, 3 fat
Glazed	4	300	15	5	7	0	10	210	38	2	3	2 1/2 carb, 1 1/2 fat
Glazed Cake	4	300	15	5	7	0	10	210	38	1	3	2 1/2 carb, 1 1/2 fat
Glazed Chocolate Cake	4	300	15	5	7	0	10	290	38	1	3	2 1/2 carb, 1 1/2 fat
✔Jelly Filled	5	240	8	3	3.5	0	0	280	37	1	3	2 1/2 carb, 1 1/2 fat
Plain Cake	4	230	15	6	7	0	10	210	21	1	3	1 1/2 carb, 3 fat

Item												Exchanges/Choices
Powdered Cake	4	260	15	5	7	0	10	210	29	2	3	2 carb, 3 fat
✔Sugar Raised	5	190	8	4	3.5	0	0	270	26	1	3	1 1/2 carb, 1 fat

PERSONAL PIZZA

✔Cheese	1	400	19	4	10	0	25	820	46	2	18	3 starch, 1 high-fat meat, 3 fat
✔Pepperoni	1	410	19	4	9	0	35	960	45	2	19	3 starch, 1 high-fat meat, 2 fat

SALADS

Caesar Salad	1	390	33	8	7	0	35	980	14	3	10	3 veg, 6 fat
Chicken Caesar	1	520	36	6	8	0	85	152	16	3	34	1/2 starch, 2 veg, 4 lean meat, 5 fat
Garden Salad	1	240	12	5	5	0	30	430	24	5	12	4 veg, 2 1/2 fat
Mediterranean Salad	1	220	11	5	4	0	15	760	23	5	10	4 veg, 2 fat

(Continued)

✔ = Healthiest Bets

SALADS *(Continued)*	Amount	Cal.	Fat (g)	% Cal. Fat	Sat. Fat (g)	Trans Fat (g)	Chol. (mg)	Sod. (mg)	Carb. (g)	Fiber (g)	Pro. (g)	Choices/Exchanges
Oriental Salad	1	580	35	5	5	1	45	1510	39	4	30	1 starch, 4 veg, 3 medium-fat meat, 4 fat
SMOOTHIE												
Mango Passion Fruit	24 oz	550	4	1	2.5	0	10	180	118	3	10	7 1/2 carb
Strawberry Banana	24 oz	550	4	1	2.5	0	10	180	118	3	10	7 1/2 carb
Wildberry	24 oz	550	4	1	2.5	0	10	180	118	2	10	7 1/2 carb
SOUPS												
Broccoli and Cheese	1 cup	180	13	7	8	0	40	1310	10	1	7	1 starch, 1 medium-fat meat, 1 1/2 fat
✔ Chicken Noodle	1 cup	140	4	3	1	0	45	840	20	1	8	1 starch, 1 lean meat
Clam Chowder	1 cup	230	11	4	4	0	30	990	20	1	10	1 starch, 1 milk, 2 fat
Lasagna Soup	1 cup	250	13	5	5	0	35	810	21	2	11	1 1/2 starch, 1 lean meat, 2 fat

✓Timberline Chili w/ Beans	1 cup	230	8	3	3	0	35	890	26	8	15	1 starch, 2 veg, 1 lean meat
STICKS												
Cinnamon Cake	1	340	20	5	10	0	15	290	37	2	4	2 1/2 carb, 4 fat
Glazed Cake	1	360	20	5	10	0	15	280	41	2	4	3 carb, 4 fat
Glazed Chocolate	1	370	21	5	10	0	0	390	41	2	3	3 carb, 4 fat
Jelly	1	420	20	4	10	0	15	310	53	2	4	3 1/2 carb, 4 fat
Plain Cake	1	310	20	6	10	0	15	250	29	2	4	2 carb, 4 fat
Powdered Cake	1	340	20	5	10	0	15	280	37	2	4	2 1/2 carb, 4 fat

✓ = Healthiest Bets

KFC
(www.kfc.com)

Light 'n Lean Choice

Original Drumsticks *(2)*
Corn on the Cob *(large, 5 1/2")*
Green Beans

Calories	460	Cholesterol (mg)	135
Fat (g)	21	Sodium (mg)	712
% calories from fat	41	Carbohydrate (g)	37
Saturated fat (g)	5	Fiber (g)	9
Trans fat (g)	0	Protein (g)	31

Exchanges: 2 starch, 1 veg, 3 lean meat, 2 fat

Healthy 'n Hearty Choice

Original Chicken Breast
BBQ Beans
Macaroni and Cheese

Calories	760	Cholesterol (mg)	130
Fat (g)	30	Sodium (mg)	2,550
% calories from fat	36	Carbohydrate (g)	70
Saturated fat (g)	9	Fiber (g)	7
Trans fat (g)	1	Protein (g)	51

Exchanges: 4 1/2 starch, 5 lean meat, 3 fat

KFC

CHICKEN

	Amount	Cal.	Fat (g)	% Cal. Fat	Sat. Fat (g)	Trans Fat (g)	Chol. (mg)	Sod. (mg)	Carb. (g)	Fiber (g)	Pro. (g)	Choices/Exchanges
✓ Breast	1	360	21	5	5	0	115	1020	7	0	37	1/2 starch, 5 lean meat, 1 fat
✓ Breast - no skin or breading	1	140	2	1	0	0	656	520	1	0	29	3 lean meat
✓ Drumstick	1	130	8	6	2	0	65	350	2	0	12	2 lean meat, 1/2 fat
Extra Crispy - Breast	1	440	27	6	6	0	105	970	15	0	34	1 starch, 4 lean meat, 2 1/2 fat
Extra Crispy - Drumstick	1	160	10	6	2	0	55	370	6	0	12	1/2 starch, 2 lean meat, 1 fat
Extra Crispy - Thigh	1	370	28	7	6	0	85	850	12	0	18	1 starch, 2 lean meat, 4 1/2 fat

(Continued)

✓ = Healthiest Bets

CHICKEN (Continued)	Amount	Cal.	Fat (g)	% Cal. Fat	Sat. Fat (g)	Trans Fat (g)	Chol. (mg)	Sod. (mg)	Carb. (g)	Fiber (g)	Pro. (g)	Choices/Exchanges
Extra Crispy - Whole Wing	1	170	11	6	2.5	0	55	350	6	1	12	1/2 starch, 2 lean meat, 1 1/2 fat
Thigh	1	330	24	7	6	0	110	870	8	0	20	1/2 starch, 3 lean meat, 3 fat
Whole Wing	1	130	8	6	2	0	50	350	4	0	11	1/2 starch, 1 lean meat, 1/2 fat
DESSERTS												
Apple Pie Mini's	3	370	20	5	6	0	0	260	44	2	2	3 carb, 3 1/2 fat
Double Chocolate Chip Cake	1 srvg	330	16	4	4	1	50	260	41	1	4	2 1/2 carb, 2 1/2 fat
Lil' Bucket Chocolate Crème	1 srvg	280	13	4	9	1	0	230	38	3	3	2 1/2 carb, 2 fat
Lil' Bucket Lemon Crème	1 srvg	410	15	3	7	1.5	0	270	61	2	7	4 carb, 2 1/2 fat

Item	Amount	Cal	Fat (g)	% Cal Fat	Sat Fat (g)	Trans Fat (g)	Chol (mg)	Sod (mg)	Carb (g)	Fiber (g)	Pro (g)	Servings/Exchanges
Lil' Bucket Strawberry Short Cake	1 srvg	210	7	30	5	0	10	125	33	1	2	2 carb, 1 1/2 fat
✓ Sweet Life Chocolate Chip Cookie	1	160	7	39	3.5	0	10	95	23	1	2	1 1/2 carb, 1 1/2 fat
✓ Sweet Life Oatmeal Raisin Cookie	1	150	5	30	2.5	0	5	135	24	1	2	1 1/2 carb, 1 fat
✓ Sweet Life Sugar Cookie	1	160	6	34	2.5	0	5	120	13	0	2	1 carb, 1 1/2 fat
✓ Teddy Grahams - Cinnamon	1 srvg	90	3	30	0.5	0	0	95	15	1	1	1 carb, 1/2 fat
POPCORN CHICKEN												
Popcorn Chicken	individ	400	26	59	4.5	0	60	1160	22	3	21	1 1/2 starch, 2 lean meat, 4 fat
✓ Popcorn Chicken	kid's	290	19	59	3.5	0	40	850	16	2	16	1 starch, 2 lean meat, 2 1/2 fat
Popcorn Chicken	lg	550	35	57	6	0	80	1600	30	3	29	2 starch, 3 lean meat, 5 fat

✓ = Healthiest Bets

(Continued)

	Amount	Cal.	Fat (g)	% Cal. Fat	Sat. Fat (g)	Trans Fat (g)	Chol. (mg)	Sod. (mg)	Carb. (g)	Fiber (g)	Pro. (g)	Choices/Exchanges
POT PIE/BOWLS												
Chicken and Biscuit Bowl	1	870	44	5	11	4.5	60	2420	88	7	29	6 starch, 2 lean meat, 7 1/2 fat
Chicken Pot Pie	1	770	40	5	15	14	115	1680	70	5	33	4 1/2 starch, 3 lean meat, 6 1/2 fat
Mashed Potato w/ Gravy Bowl	1	740	35	4	9	1.5	60	2350	80	7	27	5 1/2 starch, 2 lean meat, 5 fat
Rice w/ Gravy Bowl	1	620	28	4	7	1	60	2150	67	6	26	4 1/2 starch, 2 lean meat, 4 fat
SALADS & MORE												
✔Caesar Side Salad - no dressing or croutons	1	50	3	5	2	0	10	135	2	1	4	1 veg, 1 fat
Creamy Parmesan Caesar Dressing	1 srvg	260	26	9	5	0	15	540	4	0	2	1/2 carb, 5 fat

	Amount	Cal.	Fat (g)	Fat Cal.	Sat. Fat (g)	Trans Fat (g)	Chol. (mg)	Sod. (mg)	Carb. (g)	Fiber (g)	Pro. (g)	Choices/Exchanges
Crispy BLT Salad - no dressing	1	330	17	5	4	0	65	1130	18	1	28	1/2 starch, 1 veg, 3 lean meat, 2 fat
Crispy Caesar Salad - no dressing or croutons	1	350	19	5	6	0	70	1080	16	3	29	1/2 starch, 1 veg, 4 lean meat, 2 fat
✔Golden Italian Dressing	1 srvg	45	3	6	0	0	0	660	6	0	0	1/2 carb, 1/2 fat
✔House Side Salad - no dressing	1	15	0	0	0	0	0	10	2	1	1	Free
Original Ranch Dressing	1 srvg	200	20	9	3	0	25	470	3	0	1	4 fat
✔Original Ranch Fat Free Dressing	1 srvg	35	0	0	0	0	0	410	8	0	1	1/2 carb
✔Parmesan Garlic Croutons	1 srvg	60	3	5	0	0	0	135	8	0	2	1 carb
✔Roasted BLT Salad - no dressing	1	200	6	3	2	0	65	880	8	4	29	1 veg, 3 lean meat, 1 fat
✔Roasted Caesar Salad - no dressing & croutons	1	220	8	3	3	4.5	0	70	830	6	3	30	1 veg, 4 lean meat, 2 fat

(Continued)

✔ = Healthiest Bets

SANDWICHES AND WRAPS

	Amount	Cal.	Fat (g)	% Cal. Fat	Sat. Fat (g)	Trans Fat (g)	Chol. (mg)	Sod. (mg)	Carb. (g)	Fiber (g)	Pro. (g)	Choices/Exchanges
Crispy Twister	1	550	28	5	6	0	55	1500	49	3	26	3 1/2 starch, 2 lean meat, 4 fat
Double Crunch Sandwich	1	470	23	4	4.5	0	55	1190	38	2	27	2 1/2 starch, 3 lean meat, 3 fat
✔KFC Snacker	1	290	13	4	2.5	0	30	680	29	2	15	2 starch, 1 lean meat, 2 fat
KFC Snacker - Buffalo	1	260	8	3	1.5	0	25	860	31	1	15	2 starch, 1 lean meat, 1 fat
KFC Snacker - Fish	1	330	15	4	3	0	60	710	31	1	17	2 starch, 2 lean meat, 2 fat
KFC Snacker - Fish w/out sauce	1	290	12	4	2.5	0	60	610	29	1	17	2 starch, 2 lean meat, 1 1/2 fat

	Amount	Cal	Fat				Chol	Sod	Carb			Exchanges
KFC Snacker - Honey BBQ	1	210	3	1	0.5	0	40	530	32	2	14	2 starch, 1 lean meat
KFC Snacker - Ultimate Cheese	1	280	11	4	2.5	0.5	25	780	30	1	15	2 starch, 1 lean meat, 1 1/2 fat
Oven Roasted Twister	1	420	17	4	4	0	60	1250	40	3	28	2 1/2 starch, 3 lean meat, 1 1/2 fat
Oven Roasted Twister - no sauce	1	330	7	2	2.5	0	50	2230	39	3	28	2 1/2 starch, 3 lean meat
Tender Roast Sandwich	1	380	13	3	3	0	80	1180	29	2	37	2 starch, 4 lean meat
Tender Roast Sandwich - no sauce	1	300	5	2	1.5	0	70	1060	28	2	37	2 starch, 4 lean meat
✔Toasted Wrap w/ Crispy Strip	1	350	19	5	5	0	40	880	29	1	16	2 starch, 1 lean meat, 3 fat
✔Toasted Wrap w/ Tender Roast Fillet	1	310	15	4	5	0	50	880	24	1	21	1 1/2 starch, 2 lean meat, 1 1/2 fat

✔ = Healthiest Bets

(Continued)

	Amount	Cal.	Fat (g)	% Cal. Fat	Sat. Fat (g)	Trans Fat (g)	Chol. (mg)	Sod. (mg)	Carb. (g)	Fiber (g)	Pro. (g)	Choices/Exchanges
SIDES (INDIVIDUAL)												
Baked Beans	1 srvg	220	1	0	0	0	0	730	45	7	8	3 starch
Biscuit	1 srvg	220	11	5	2.5	3.5	0	640	24	1	4	2 starch, 2 fat
Cole Slaw	1 srvg	180	10	5	1.5	0	5	270	22	3	1	1 starch, 1 1/2 fat
✓Corn on the Cob	3"	70	5	6	0.5	0	0	5	13	3	2	1 starch, 1/2 fat
Corn on the Cob	5.5"	150	3	2	1	0	0	10	26	7	5	2 starch, 1/2 fat
✓Green Beans	1 srvg	50	2	4	0	0	5	2	7	2	2	1 veg, 1/2 fat
Macaroni & Cheese	1 srvg	180	8	4	3.5	1	15	800	18	0	6	1 starch, 2 fat
✓Mashed Potatoes - no gravy	1 srvg	110	4	3	1	0	0	320	17	1	2	1 starch, 1 fat
✓Mashed Potatoes w/ Gravy	1 srvg	140	5	3	1	0.5	0	560	20	1	2	1 starch, 1 fat

	Amount	Cal	Fat (g)	% Cal. Fat	Sat. Fat (g)	Trans Fat (g)	Chol. (mg)	Sod. (mg)	Carb. (g)	Fiber (g)	Pro. (g)	Exchanges/Choices
Potato Salad	1 srvg	180	9	5	1.5	0	5	470	22	2	2	1 starch, 2 fat
Potato Wedges	1 srvg	260	13	5	2.5	0	0	740	33	3	4	2 starch, 2 fat
Seasoned Rice	1 srvg	150	4	2	0	0	0	630	32	2	4	2 starch, 1/2 fat
STRIPS												
Crispy Strips	3	350	19	5	3.5	0	70	1190	16	0	29	1 starch, 4 lean meat, 1 1/2 fat
Crispy Strips	2	240	13	5	2.5	0	50	800	11	0	20	1/2 starch, 3 lean meat, 1 fat
WINGS												
Boneless Fiery Buffalo	5	420	20	4	3.5	0	65	2260	33	3	28	2 starch, 3 lean meat, 2 fat
Boneless Honey BBQ	5	450	20	4	3.5	0	65	1880	41	4	28	2 1/2 starch, 3 lean meat, 2 1/2 fat
Boneless Sweet & Spicy	5	440	19	4	3.5	0	65	1700	38	3	27	2 1/2 starch, 3 lean meat, 2 fat

(Continued)

✔ = Healthiest Bets

WINGS *(Continued)*	Amount	Cal.	Fat (g)	% Cal. Fat	Sat. Fat (g)	Trans Fat (g)	Chol. (mg)	Sod. (mg)	Carb. (g)	Fiber (g)	Pro. (g)	Choices/Exchanges
Boneless Teriyaki	5	500	21	4	3.5	0	65	1730	50	3	28	3 1/2 starch, 3 lean meat, 2 1/2 fat
Fiery Buffalo	5	380	24	6	5	0	105	1480	19	2	21	1 1/2 starch, 2 lean meat, 3 1/2 fat
Honey BBQ	5	390	24	6	5	0	105	830	23	3	21	1 1/2 starch, 2 lean meat, 3 1/2 fat
Hot	5	350	24	6	5	0	105	740	14	2	20	1 starch, 2 lean meat, 3 1/2 fat
Sweet & Spicy	5	400	24	5	5	0	105	760	24	2	21	1 1/2 starch, 2 lean meat, 3 1/2 fat
Teriyaki	5	480	25	5	5	0	105	830	40	2	22	2 1/2 starch, 2 lean meat, 4 fat

✔ = Healthiest Bets

McDonald's
(www.mcdonalds.com)

Light 'n Lean Choice

Premium Asian Salad with Grilled Chicken
Newman's Own Low-Fat Balsamic
Vinaigrette *(1.5 oz, 3 Tbsp)*
Fruit and Yogurt Parfait with granola

Calories	500	Cholesterol (mg)	70
Fat (g)	15	Sodium (mg)	1,705
% calories from fat	27	Carbohydrate (g)	58
Saturated fat (g)	2	Fiber (g)	6
Trans fat (g)	0	Protein (g)	36

Exchanges: 2 veg, 1/2 starch, 1 1/2 carb, 1 fruit, 3 lean meat, 1 fat

Healthy 'n Hearty Choice

Hamburger
French Fries *(small)*
Premium Southwest Salad (no chicken) with
Newman's Own Low-Fat Family Italian
Recipe *(1.5 oz, 3 Tbsp)*

Calories	660	Cholesterol (mg)	35
Fat (g)	26	Sodium (mg)	1,310
% calories from fat	35	Carbohydrate (g)	86
Saturated fat (g)	7	Fiber (g)	11
Trans fat (g)	1	Protein (g)	22

Exchanges: 4 starch, 1 carb, 2 veg, 1 medium-fat meat, 4 fat

McDonald's

BREAKFAST

	Amount	Cal.	Fat (g)	% Cal. Fat	Sat. Fat (g)	Trans Fat (g)	Chol. (mg)	Sod. (mg)	Carb. (g)	Fiber (g)	Pro. (g)	Choices/Exchanges
Bacon, Egg & Cheese Biscuit	reg	430	24	5	12	0	240	1230	37	2	16	2 1/2 starch, 1 medium-fat meat, 3 1/2 fat
Bacon, Egg & Cheese Biscuit	lg	520	30	5	13	0	256	1520	43	3	19	3 starch, 1 medium-fat meat, 4 1/2 fat
Bacon, Egg & Cheese McGriddles	1	420	19	4	9	0	240	1190	48	2	16	3 starch, 1 medium-fat meat, 3 fat
Big Breakfast, large biscuit	1	800	52	6	18	0	555	1680	56	4	28	3 1/2 starch, 2 medium-fat meat, 8 fat
Big Breakfast, regular biscuit	1	740	48	6	17	0	555	1560	51	3	28	3 1/2 starch, 3 medium-fat meat, 7 fat

Item	Amount	Cal.	Fat (g)	% Cal. Fat	Sat. Fat (g)	Trans Fat (g)	Chol. (mg)	Sod. (mg)	Carb. (g)	Fiber (g)	Pro. (g)	Servings/Exchanges
Biscuit	reg	260	12	4	7	0		740	33	2	5	2 carb, 2 1/2 fat
Biscuit	lg	320	16	5	8	0		850	39	3	5	2 1/2 carb, 3 fat
Deluxe Breakfast - reg biscuit, no syrup or margarine	1	1090	56	5	19	0	575	2150	111	6	36	7 1/2 starch, 2 medium-fat meat, 8 fat
Deluxe Breakfast, lg biscuit, no syrup or margarine	1	1150	60	5	20	0	575	2260	116	7	36	7 1/2 starch, 2 medium-fat meat, 9 fat
✔Egg McMuffin	1	300	12	4	5	0	260	820	30	2	18	2 starch, 2 medium-fat meat, 1/2 fat
✔English Muffin	1	160	3	2	0.5	0	0	280	27	2	5	2 carb, 1/2 fat
✔Grape Jam	.5 oz	35	0	0	0	0	0	0	9	0	0	1/2 carb
✔Hash Brown	1	150	9	5	1.5	0	0	310	15	2	1	1 starch, 2 fat
Hotcake syrup	1 pkg	180	0	0	0	0	0	20	45	0	0	3 carb
Hotcakes - no syrup or margarine	1 order	350	9	2	2	0	20	590	60	3	8	4 starch, 2 fat

(Continued)

✔ = Healthiest Bets

BREAKFAST *(Continued)*	Amount	Cal.	Fat (g)	% Cal. Fat	Sat. Fat (g)	Trans Fat (g)	Chol. (mg)	Sod. (mg)	Carb. (g)	Fiber (g)	Pro. (g)	Choices/Exchanges
Hotcakes and Sausage - no syrup or margarine	1 order	520	24	4	7	0	50	930	61	3	15	4 starch, 2 high-fat meat, 1 fat
McSkillet Burrito w/ Sausage	1	610	36	5	14	0.5	410	1390	44	3	27	3 starch, 3 medium-fat meat, 4 1/2 fat
McSkillet Burrito w/ Steak	1	570	30	5	12	1	430	1470	44	3	32	3 starch, 3 medium-fat meat, 2 1/2 fat
Sausage Biscuit	reg	410	20	4	8	0	30	1180	41	2	17	2 1/2 starch, 1 medium-fat meat, 2 1/2 fat
Sausage Biscuit	lg	480	31	6	13	0	30	1190	39	3	11	2 1/2 starch, 5 1/2 fat
Sausage Biscuit w/ Egg	reg	430	27	6	12	0	30	1080	34	2	11	2 1/2 starch, 1 medium-fat meat, 5 fat
Sausage Biscuit w/ Egg	lg	570	37	6	15	0	250	1280	42	3	18	3 starch, 1 medium-fat meat, 6 fat
✔Sausage Burrito	1	300	16	5	7	0.5	130	830	26	1	12	1 1/2 starch, 2 high-fat meat, 1/2 fat

	Amount	Cal.	Fat	Sat. Fat			Chol.	Sod.	Carb.	Fiber	Pro.	Exchanges/Choices
Sausage McGriddles	1	420	22	5	8	0	35	1030	44	2	11	3 starch, 4 fat
Sausage McMuffin	1	370	22	5	8	0	45	850	29	2	14	2 starch, 1 medium-fat meat, 3 fat
Sausage McMuffin w/ Egg	1	450	27	5	40	0	285	920	30	2	21	2 starch, 2 medium-fat meat, 3 1/2 fat
Sausage Patty	1	170	15	8	5	0	30	340	1	0	7	1 high-fat meat, 1 fat
Sausage, Egg & Cheese McGriddles	1	560	32	12	12	0	265	1360	48	2	20	3 starch, 1 medium-fat meat, 5 fat
✔Scrambled Eggs - 2	1 order	170	11	6	4	0	520	180	1	0	15	2 medium-fat meat
Southern Style Chicken Biscuit	reg	410	20	4	8	0	30	1180	41	2	17	2 1/2 starch, 1 lean meat, 3 fat
Southern Style Chicken Biscuit	lg	470	24	5	9	0	30	1290	46	3	17	3 starch, 1 lean meat, 4 fat
✔Strawberry Preserves	.5 oz	35	0	0	0	0	0	0	9	0	0	1/2 carb
✔Whipped Margarine	1 pat	40	5	1.5	0	0	0	55	0	0	0	1 fat

✔ = Healthiest Bets

(Continued)

	Amount	Cal.	Fat (g)	% Cal. Fat	Sat. Fat (g)	Trans Fat (g)	Chol. (mg)	Sod. (mg)	Carb. (g)	Fiber (g)	Pro. (g)	Choices/Exchanges
CHICKEN MCNUGGET AND SELECTS SAUCES												
✔Barbeque Sauce	1 oz	50	0	0	0	0	0	260	12	0	0	1 starch
Creamy Ranch Sauce	1.5 oz	200	22	10	3.4	0	10	320	2	0	0	4.4 fat
✔Honey	1 oz	50	0	0	0	0	0	260	12	0	0	1 starch
✔Hot Mustard	1 oz	60	2.5	4	0	0	5	250	9	2	1	1/2 starch, 1/2 fat
✔Southwestern Chipotle Barbeque Sauce	1.5 oz	70	0	0	0	0	0	260	18	1	0	1 starch
Spicy Buffalo Sauce	1.5 oz	70	7	9	1	0	0	960	1	2	0	1.4 fat
✔Sweet 'N Sour Sauce	1 oz	50	0	0	0	0	0	150	12	0	0	1 starch
✔Tangy Honey Mustard	1.5 oz	70	2.5	3	0	0	5	170	13	0	1	1 starch, 1/2 fat
CHICKEN MCNUGGETS & SELECTS STRIPS												
✔Chicken McNuggets	6 pcs	280	17	5	3	0	40	600	16	0	14	1 starch, 2 lean meat, 2 1/2 fat

	Amount	Cal.	Fat (g)	% Cal. Fat	Sat. Fat (g)	Trans Fat (g)	Chol. (mg)	Sod. (mg)	Carb. (g)	Fiber (g)	Pro. (g)	Servings/Exchanges
✓ Chicken McNuggets	4 pcs	190	12	57	2	0	30	400	11	0	10	1/2 starch, 1 lean meat, 1 1/2 fat
Chicken McNuggets	10 pcs	460	29	57	5	0	70	1000	27	0	24	2 starch, 3 lean meat, 4 fat
Chicken Selects Premium Breast Strips	3 pcs	400	24	54	3.5	0	50	1010	23	0	23	1 1/2 starch, 3 lean meat, 3 fat
Chicken Selects Premium Breast Strips	5 pcs	660	40	55	6	0	85	1680	39	0	37	2 1/2 starch, 4 lean meat, 5 1/2 fat
DESSERTS AND SHAKES												
✓ Apple Dippers	1 order	35	0	0	0	0	0	0	8	0	0	1/2 fruit
Baked Apple Pie	1	270	12	40	3.5	5	0	190	36	4	3	2 1/2 carb, 2 1/2 fat
✓ Chocolate Chip Cookie	1	160	7	39	2.5	1.5	10	90	22	1	2	1 1/2 carb, 1 1/2 fat
Chocolate Triple Thick Shake	21 oz	770	18	21	11	1	70	330	134	1	18	9 carb, 3 fat
Chocolate Triple Thick Shake	16 oz	580	14	22	8	1	50	250	102	1	13	7 carb, 2 fat

✓ = Healthiest Bets

(Continued)

DESSERTS AND SHAKES *(Continued)*	Amount	Cal.	Fat (g)	% Cal. Fat	Sat. Fat (g)	Trans Fat (g)	Chol. (mg)	Sod. (mg)	Carb. (g)	Fiber (g)	Pro. (g)	Choices/Exchanges
Chocolate Triple Thick Shake	12 oz	440	10	2	6	0.5	40	190	76	1	10	5 carb, 2 fat
Chocolate Triple Thick Shake	32 oz	1160	27	2	16	2	100	510	203	2	27	13 1/2 carb, 4 fat
Cinnamon Melts	1 order	460	19	4	9	0	15	370	66	3	6	4 1/2 carb, 3 fat
✔Fruit and Yogurt Parfait	1	160	2	1	1	0	5	85	31	1	4	1 carb, 1 milk
✔Fruit and Yogurt Parfait - no Granola	1	130	2	1	1	0	5	55	25	0	4	1/2 carb, 1 milk
Hot Caramel Sundae	1	340	8	2	5	0	30	160	60	1	7	4 carb, 1 1/2 fat
Hot Fudge Sundae	1	330	10	3	7	0	25	180	54	2	8	3 1/2 carb, 2 fat
✔Kiddie Cone	1	45	1	2	0.5	0	5	20	8	0	1	1/2 carb
✔Low Fat Caramel Dip	1 order	70	1	1	0	0	5	35	15	0	0	1 carb
McDonaldland Cookies	1 pkg	250	8	3	2	0	0	260	42	1	4	3 carb, 1 1/2 fat

Item	Amount											
McFlurry w/ M&M's Candies	12 oz	620	20	3	12	1	55	190	96	1	14	6 1/2 carb, 3 1/2 fat
McFlurry w/ Oreo Cookies	12 oz	550	17	3	9	1	50	250	88	1	13	6 carb, 3 fat
✔ Oatmeal Raisin Cookie	1	150	6	4	1.5	1.5	10	135	22	1	2	1 1/2 carb, 1 fat
✔ Peanuts (for Sundaes)	1 pkg	45	4	8	0.5	0	0	0	2	1	2	1 fat
Strawberry Sundae	1	280	6	2	4	0	25	95	49	1	6	3 1/2 carb, 1 fat
Strawberry Triple Thick Shake	12 oz	420	10	2	6	0.5	40	130	73	0	10	5 carb, 2 fat
Strawberry Triple Thick Shake	16 oz	560	13	2	8	1	50	170	97	0	13	6 1/2 carb, 2 fat
Strawberry Triple Thick Shake	21 oz	740	18	2	11	1	70	230	128	0	17	8 1/2 carb, 3 fat
Strawberry Triple Thick Shake	32 oz	1110	26	2	16	2	100	350	194	0	25	13 carb, 4 fat

✔ = Healthiest Bets

(Continued)

DESSERTS AND SHAKES *(Continued)*	Amount	Cal.	Fat (g)	% Cal. Fat	Sat. Fat (g)	Trans Fat (g)	Chol. (mg)	Sod. (mg)	Carb. (g)	Fiber (g)	Pro. (g)	Choices/Exchanges
✔Sugar Cookie	1	150	6	4	1.5	2	5	110	21	0	2	1 1/2 carb, 1 fat
✔Vanilla Reduced Fat Ice Cream Cone	1	150	4	2	2	0	15	60	24	0	4	1 1/2 carb, 1/2 fat
Vanilla Triple Thick Shake	12 oz	420	10	2	6	0.5	40	140	72	0	9	5 carb, 1 1/2 fat
Vanilla Triple Thick Shake	16 oz	550	13	2	8	1	50	190	96	0	13	6 1/2 carb, 2 fat
Vanilla Triple Thick Shake	21 oz	740	18	2	11	1	70	250	128	0	17	8 1/2 carb, 3 fat
Vanilla Triple Thick Shake	32 oz	1110	26	2	16	2	100	370	193	0	25	13 carb, 4 fat
FRENCH FRIES												
French Fries	sm	230	11	4	1.5	0	0	160	29	3	3	2 starch, 2 fat
French Fries	med	380	19	5	2.5	0	0	270	48	5	4	3 starch, 4 fat
French Fries	lg	500	25	5	3.5	0	0	350	63	6	6	4 starch, 4 1/2 fat
ICED COFFEE												
✔Caramel Iced Coffee	16 oz	130	5	3	3.5	0	20	80	21	0	1	1 1/2 carb, 1 fat

	Serving	Calories										Exchanges/Choices
Caramel Iced Coffee	22 oz	190	8	4	5	0	30	115	27	0	1	2 carb, 1 1/2 fat
Caramel Iced Coffee	32 oz	270	11	4	7	0	40	160	41	0	2	2 1/2 carb, 1 1/2 fat
✔ Hazelnut Iced Coffee	16 oz	130	5	3	3.5	0	20	40	21	0	1	1 1/2 carb, 1 1/2 fat
Hazelnut Iced Coffee	22 oz	190	8	4	5	0	30	60	29	0	1	2 carb, 1 1/2 fat
Hazelnut Iced Coffee	32 oz	270	11	4	7	0	40	80	43	0	2	3 carb, 1 1/2 fat
✔ Regular Iced Coffee	16 oz	140	5	3	3.5	0	20	40	22	0	1	1 1/2 carb, 1 fat
Regular Iced Coffee	22 oz	200	8	4	5	0	30	60	30	0	1	2 carb, 1 1/2 fat
Regular Iced Coffee	32 oz	280	11	4	7	0	40	80	45	0	2	3 carb, 1 1/2 fat
✔ Sugar Free Vanilla Iced Coffee	16 oz	60	5	8	3.5	0	20	70	8	0	1	1/2 carb
Sugar Free Vanilla Iced Coffee	22 oz	90	8	8	5	0	30	95	11	0	1	1/2 carb
Sugar Free Vanilla Iced Coffee	32 oz	120	11	8	7	0	40	140	16	0	2	1 carb

(Continued)

✔ = Healthiest Bets

ICED COFFEE *(Continued)*	Amount	Cal.	Fat (g)	% Cal. Fat	Sat. Fat (g)	Trans Fat (g)	Chol. (mg)	Sod. (mg)	Carb. (g)	Fiber (g)	Pro. (g)	Choices/Exchanges
✔Vanilla Iced Coffee	16 oz	130	5	3	3.5	0	20	40	21	0	1	1 1/2 carb, 1 fat
Vanilla Iced Coffee	22 oz	190	8	4	5	0	30	60	29	0	1	2 carb, 1 1/2 fat
Vanilla Iced Coffee	32 oz	270	11	4	7	0	40	80	43	0	2	3 carb, 1 1/2 fat
SALAD DRESSING												
✔Newman's Own Creamy Caesar Dressing	2 oz	190	18	9	2.4	0	20	500	4	0	2	1/2 carb, 3 1/2 fat
✔Newman's Own Creamy Southwest Dressing	1.5 oz	100	6	5	1	0	20	340	11	0	1	1/2 carb, 1 fat
✔Newman's Own Low Fat Balsamic Vinaigrette	1.5 oz	40	3	7	0	0	0	730	4	0	0	1/2 carb, 1/2 fat
✔Newman's Own Low Fat Family Italian Recipe	1.5 oz	60	2.5	4	0	0	0	730	8	0	1	1/2 carb, 1/2 fat
✔Newman's Own Ranch Dressing	2 oz	170	15	8	2.5	0	20	530	9	0	1	1/2 carb, 3 fat

SALADS

	Amount	Cal	Fat (g)	% Cal Fat	Sat. Fat (g)	Trans Fat (g)	Chol (mg)	Sod (mg)	Carb (g)	Fiber (g)	Pro (g)	Servings/Exchanges
✔ Butter Garlic Croutons	.5 oz	60	1.5	23	0	0	0	140	10	1	2	1/2 starch
✔ Premium Asian Salad - no Chicken	1	150	7	42	0.5	0	0	35	15	5	8	1 starch, 1 1/2 fat
✔ Premium Asian Salad w/ Crispy Chicken	1	410	20	44	2.5	0	45	850	31	5	28	1 starch, 3 veg, 3 lean meat, 2 fat
✔ Premium Asian Salad w/ Grilled Chicken	1	300	10	30	1	0	65	890	23	5	32	1/2 starch, 3 veg, 3 lean meat
✔ Premium Bacon Ranch Salad w/ Crispy Chicken	1	370	20	49	6	0	75	970	20	3	29	3 veg, 4 lean meat, 1 1/2 fat
✔ Premium Bacon Ranch Salad w/ Grilled Chicken	1	260	9	31	4	0	90	1010	12	3	33	3 veg, 4 lean meat
✔ Premium Bacon Salad - no Chicken	1	140	7	45	3.5	0	25	300	10	3	9	2 veg, 1 medium-fat meat
✔ Premium Caesar Salad - no Chicken	1	90	4	40	2.5	0	10	180	9	3	7	3 veg, 1/2 fat

✔ = Healthiest Bets

(Continued)

SALADS *(Continued)*	Amount	Cal.	Fat (g)	% Cal. Fat	Sat. Fat (g)	Trans Fat (g)	Chol. (mg)	Sod. (mg)	Carb. (g)	Fiber (g)	Pro. (g)	Choices/Exchanges
✔Premium Caesar Salad w/ Crispy Chicken	1	330	17	5	4.5	0	60	840	20	3	26	3 veg, 3 lean meat, 1 1/2 fat
✔Premium Caesar Salad w/ Grilled Chicken	1	220	6	2	3	0	75	890	12	3	30	3 veg, 3 lean meat
✔Premium Southwest Salad - no Chicken	1	140	4.5	3	2	0	10	150	20	6	6	4 veg, 1 medium-fat meat
✔Premium Southwest Salad w/ Crispy Chicken	1	430	20	4	4	0	55	920	38	6	26	1 starch, 3 veg, 3 lean meat, 2 fat
✔Premium Southwest Salad w/ Grilled Chicken	1	320	9	3	3	0	70	960	30	6	30	1 starch, 3 veg, 3 lean meat
✔Side Salad	1	20	0	0	0	0	0	10	4	1	1	1 veg
Snack Size Fruit and Walnut Salad	1	210	8	3	1.5	0	5	60	31	2	4	2 fruit, 1 1/2 fat

SANDWICHES

Item		Cal								Exchanges
Big Mac	1	540	29	5	10	1.5	75	1040	45	3	25	3 starch, 2 medium-fat meat, 3 1/2 fat
Big N' Tasty	1	460	24	5	8	1.5	70	710	37	3	24	2 1/2 starch, 2 medium-fat meat, 2 1/2 fat
Big N' Tasty w/ Cheese	1	510	28	5	11	1.5	85	960	38	3	27	2 1/2 starch, 3 medium-fat meat, 3 fat
✔Cheeseburger	1	300	12	4	6	0.5	40	750	33	2	15	2 starch, 1 medium-fat meat, 1 fat
✔Chipotle BBQ Snack Wrap (Crispy)	1	330	15	4	4.5	0	30	810	35	1	14	2 1/2 starch, 1 lean meat, 2 1/2 fat
✔Chipotle BBQ Snack Wrap (Grilled)	1	260	9	3	3.5	0	45	830	28	1	18	2 starch, 2 lean meat, 1/2 fat
Double Cheeseburger	1	440	23	5	11	1.5	80	1150	34	2	25	2 1/2 starch, 3 medium-fat meat, 2 fat

(Continued)

✔ = Healthiest Bets

SANDWICHES *(Continued)*	Amount	Cal.	Fat (g)	% Cal. Fat	Sat. Fat (g)	Trans Fat (g)	Chol. (mg)	Sod. (mg)	Carb. (g)	Fiber (g)	Pro. (g)	Choices/Exchanges
Double Quarter Pounder w/ Cheese	1	740	42	5	19	2.5	155	1380	40	3	48	2 1/2 starch, 6 medium-fat meat, 2 1/2 fat
Filet-O-Fish	1	380	18	4	3.5	0	40	640	38	2	15	2 1/2 starch, 1 lean meat, 3 fat
✓Hamburger	1	250	9	3	3.5	0.5	25	520	31	2	12	2 starch, 1 medium-fat meat, 1 fat
✓Honey Mustard Snack Wrap (Crispy)	1	330	16	4	4.5	0	30	780	34	1	14	2 1/2 starch, 1 lean meat, 2 1/2 fat
✓Honey Mustard Snack Wrap (Grilled)	1	260	9	3	3.5	0	45	800	27	1	18	2 starch, 2 lean meat, 1/2 fat
✓McChicken	1	360	16	4	3	0	35	830	40	2	14	2 1/2 starch, 1 lean meat, 2 1/2 fat
McRib	1	500	26	5	10	0	70	980	44	3	22	3 starch, 2 lean meat, 4 fat

Item	Serv.	Cal.	Fat									Exchanges
Premium Crispy Chicken Classic	1	530	20	3	3.5	0	50	1150	59	3	28	4 starch, 2 lean meat, 2 1/2 fat
Premium Crispy Chicken Club	1	630	28	4	7	0	75	1420	60	4	36	4 starch, 3 lean meat, 3 1/2 fat
Premium Crispy Chicken Ranch BLT	1	580	23	4	4.5	0	60	1460	61	3	32	4 starch, 3 lean meat, 3 fat
Premium Grilled Chicken Classic	1	420	10	2	2	0	70	1190	51	3	32	3 1/2 starch, 3 lean meat
Premium Grilled Chicken Club	1	530	17	3	6	0	90	1470	52	4	40	3 1/2 starch, 4 lean meat, 1 fat
Premium Grilled Chicken Ranch BLT	1	470	12	2	3	0	80	1500	53	3	36	3 1/2 starch, 4 lean meat
✓ Quarter Pounder	1	410	19	4	7	1	65	730	37	2	24	2 1/2 starch, 2 medium-fat meat, 1 1/2 fat
Quarter Pounder w/ Cheese	1	510	26	5	12	1.5	90	1190	40	3	29	2 1/2 starch, 3 medium-fat meat, 2 fat

(Continued)

✓ = Healthiest Bets

SANDWICHES *(Continued)*	Amount	Cal.	Fat (g)	% Cal. Fat	Sat. Fat (g)	Trans Fat (g)	Chol. (mg)	Sod. (mg)	Carb. (g)	Fiber (g)	Pro. (g)	Choices/Exchanges
✔Ranch Snack Wrap (Crispy)	1	340	17	5	4.5	0	30	810	33	1	14	2 starch, 1 lean meat, 3 fat
✔Ranch Snack Wrap (Grilled)	1	270	10	3	4	0	45	830	26	4	17	1 1/2 starch, 2 lean meat, 1 fat
Southern Style Crispy Chicken	1	400	17	4	3	0	45	1030	39	1	24	2 1/2 starch, 2 lean meat, 2 fat

✔ = Healthiest Bets

Papa John's Pizza
(www.papajohns.com)

Light 'n Lean Choice

14" Original-Crust Garden Fresh Pizza *(2 slices)*

Calories	560	Cholesterol (mg)	30
Fat (g)	18	Sodium (mg)	1,360
% calories from fat	29	Carbohydrate (g)	78
Saturated fat (g)	5	Fiber (g)	4
Trans fat (g)	0	Protein (g)	22

Exchanges: 5 starch, 3 1/2 fat

Healthy 'n Hearty Choice

14" Original Crust Spinach Alfredo Chicken Tomato Pizza *(3 slices)*

Calories	600	Cholesterol (mg)	50
Fat (g)	22	Sodium (mg)	1,400
% calories from fat	33	Carbohydrate (g)	74
Saturated fat (g)	9	Fiber (g)	4
Trans fat (g)	0	Protein (g)	28

Exchanges: 5 starch, 1 veg, 2 medium-fat meat, 2 fat

(Continued)

Papa John's Pizza

10" ORIGINAL CRUST PIZZAS

	Amount	Cal.	Fat (g)	% Cal. Fat	Sat. Fat (g)	Trans Fat (g)	Chol. (mg)	Sod. (mg)	Carb. (g)	Fiber (g)	Pro. (g)	Choices/Exchanges
BBQ Chicken & Bacon Pizza	1 slice	220	8	3	2.5	0	20	640	30	1	10	2 starch, 1 medium-fat meat, 1 fat
✓Cheese	1 slice	180	6	3	1.5	0	10	430	25	1	7	1 1/2 starch, 1 fat
✓Chicken Bacon Ranch	1 slice	220	10	4	2.5	0	20	470	26	1	10	1 1/2 starch, 1 medium-fat meat, 1 fat
✓Garden Fresh	1 slice	180	6	3	1.5	0	10	460	26	1	8	1 1/2 starch, 1 fat
Hawaiian BBQ Chicken	1 slice	230	8	3	2.5	0	20	640	31	1	10	2 starch, 1 medium-fat meat, 1 fat
Italian Meats Trio	1 slice	170	6	3	3	0	15	510	19	1	8	1 1/2 starch, 1 medium-fat meat, 1/2 fat

The Meats	1 slice	230	11	4	3.5	0	20	620	25	1	10	1 1/2 starch, 1 medium-fat meat, 1 1/2 fat
✔Papa's White	1 slice	190	7	3	2.5	0	15	490	25	1	8	1 1/2 starch, 1 1/2 fat
Pepperoni	1 slice	210	9	4	2.5	0	15	540	25	1	9	1 1/2 starch, 1 medium-fat meat, 1 fat
Sausage	1 slice	220	10	4	3	0	15	540	25	2	8	1 1/2 starch, 2 fat
Sicilian Classic Pizza	1 slice	240	9	3	4.5	0	20	700	26	2	10	1 1/2 starch, 1 medium-fat meat, 1 fat
Smokehouse Bacon & Ham	1 slice	220	9	4	2.5	0	20	590	26	1	10	1 1/2 starch, 1 medium-fat meat, 1 fat
Spicy Italian	1 slice	230	7	3	5	0	20	600	26	2	9	1 1/2 starch, 1 medium-fat meat, 1 fat
✔Spinach Alfredo	1 slice	190	7	3	3	0	15	420	24	1	8	1 1/2 starch, 1 1/2 fat
✔Spinach Alfredo Chicken Tomato	1 slice	200	8	4	3	0	20	470	25	1	9	1 1/2 starch, 1 medium-fat meat, 1 fat

✔ = Healthiest Bets

(Continued)

10" ORIGINAL CRUST PIZZAS *(Continued)*	Amount	Cal.	Fat (g)	% Cal. Fat	Sat. Fat (g)	Trans Fat (g)	Chol. (mg)	Sod. (mg)	Carb. (g)	Fiber (g)	Pro. (g)	Choices/Exchanges
Tuscan Six Cheese	1 slice	210	8	3	3	0	15	530	26	1	10	1 1/2 starch, 1 medium-fat meat, 1 fat
The Works	1 slice	220	8	3	4	0	15	610	26	2	9	1 1/2 starch, 1 medium-fat meat, 1 fat

12" ORIGINAL CRUST PIZZAS

10" ORIGINAL CRUST PIZZAS *(Continued)*	Amount	Cal.	Fat (g)	% Cal. Fat	Sat. Fat (g)	Trans Fat (g)	Chol. (mg)	Sod. (mg)	Carb. (g)	Fiber (g)	Pro. (g)	Choices/Exchanges
BBQ Chicken & Bacon Pizza	1 slice	240	8	3	2.5	0	20	690	32	1	11	2 starch, 1 medium-fat meat, 1 fat
Cheese	1 slice	210	8	3	2.5	0	15	510	27	1	9	2 starch, 1 medium-fat meat, 1 fat
✔ Chicken Bacon Ranch	1 slice	240	10	4	2.5	0	20	500	27	1	11	2 starch, 1 medium-fat meat, 1 fat
✔ Garden Fresh	1 slice	200	7	3	2	0	10	490	28	2	8	2 starch, 1 1/2 fat
Hawaiian BBQ Chicken	1 slice	240	8	3	2.5	0	20	690	33	1	11	2 starch, 1 medium-fat meat, 1 fat

	Amount											Exchanges/Choices
Italian Meats Trio	1 slice	250	8	3	5	0	25	740	27	2	12	2 starch, 1 medium-fat meat, 1/2 fat
The Meats	1 slice	240	11	4	3.5	0	20	640	26	1	11	1 1/2 starch, 1 medium-fat meat, 1 1/2 fat
Papa's White	1 slice	200	8	4	2.5	0	15	520	26	1	8	1 1/2 starch, 1 1/2 fat
Pepperoni	1 slice	220	9	4	3	0	15	580	26	1	9	1 1/2 starch, 1 medium-fat meat, 1 1/2 fat
Sausage	1 slice	240	11	4	3.5	0	15	580	26	2	9	1 1/2 starch, 1 medium-fat meat, 1 1/2 fat
Sicilian Classic Pizza	1 slice	260	10	3	5	0	25	770	27	2	12	2 starch, 1 medium-fat meat, 1 fat
Smokehouse Bacon & Ham	1 slice	240	9	3	3	0	20	640	27	1	11	2 starch, 1 medium-fat meat, 1 fat
Spicy Italian	1 slice	260	8	3	7	0	20	680	27	2	11	2 starch, 1 medium-fat meat, 1 fat

✔ = Healthiest Bets

12" ORIGINAL CRUST PIZZAS *(Continued)*	Amount	Cal.	Fat (g)	% Cal. Fat	Sat. Fat (g)	Trans Fat (g)	Chol. (mg)	Sod. (mg)	Carb. (g)	Fiber (g)	Pro. (g)	Choices/Exchanges
✔ Spinach Alfredo	1 slice	210	8	3	3	0	15	450	26	1	8	1 1/2 starch, 1 1/2 fat
✔ Spinach Alfredo Chicken Tomato	1 slice	220	8	3	3.5	0	20	500	26	1	10	1 1/2 starch, 1 medium-fat meat, 1 fat
Tuscan Six Cheese	1 slice	230	9	4	3.5	0	20	570	27	1	11	2 starch, 1 medium-fat meat, 1 fat
The Works	1 slice	230	8	3	3.5	0	15	610	28	2	10	2 starch, 1 medium-fat meat, 1 fat

12" PAN CRUST PIZZAS

	Amount	Cal.	Fat (g)	% Cal. Fat	Sat. Fat (g)	Trans Fat (g)	Chol. (mg)	Sod. (mg)	Carb. (g)	Fiber (g)	Pro. (g)	Choices/Exchanges
BBQ Chicken & Bacon Pizza	1 slice	430	22	5	7	0	30	940	43	1	15	3 starch, 1 medium-fat meat, 3 fat
Cheese	1 slice	410	23	5	7	0	20	750	38	1	13	2 1/2 starch, 1 medium-fat meat, 4 fat
Chicken Bacon Ranch	1 slice	430	25	5	7	0	25	680	37	1	15	2 1/2 starch, 1 medium-fat meat, 4 fat

Garden Fresh	1 slice	370	19	5	6	0	15	660	39	2	11	2 1/2 starch, 4 fat
Hawaiian BBQ Chicken	1 slice	440	22	5	7	0	30	940	45	1	15	3 starch, 1 medium-fat meat, 3 fat
Italian Meats Trio	1 slice	440	21	4	11	0	30	1040	38	2	16	2 1/2 starch, 1 medium-fat meat, 3 fat
The Meats	1 slice	440	26	5	8	0	30	890	37	1	15	2 1/2 starch, 1 medium-fat meat, 4 fat
Papa's White	1 slice	370	21	5	7	0	20	700	35	1	11	2 1/2 starch, 1 medium-fat meat, 3 fat
Pepperoni	1 slice	410	24	5	8	0	20	820	37	1	13	2 1/2 starch, 1 medium-fat meat, 4 fat
Sausage	1 slice	420	25	5	8	0	20	790	37	2	12	2 1/2 starch, 1 medium-fat meat, 4 fat
Sicilian Classic Pizza	1 slice	450	23	5	11	0	35	1040	37	2	16	2 1/2 starch, 1 medium-fat meat, 3 1/2 fat

(Continued)

✔ = Healthiest Bets

12" PAN CRUST PIZZAS *(Continued)*	Amount	Cal.	Fat (g)	% Cal. Fat	Sat. Fat (g)	Trans Fat (g)	Chol. (mg)	Sod. (mg)	Carb. (g)	Fiber (g)	Pro. (g)	Choices/Exchanges
Smokehouse Bacon & Ham	1 slice	420	23	5	7	0	30	870	38	1	15	2 1/2 starch, 1 medium-fat meat, 3 fat
Spicy Italian	1 slice	470	21	4	14	0	30	950	38	3	15	2 1/2 starch, 1 medium-fat meat, 4 fat
Spinach Alfredo	1 slice	380	22	5	8	0	20	610	35	1	12	2 1/2 starch, 1 medium-fat meat, 3 fat
Spinach Alfredo Chicken Tomato	1 slice	390	22	5	8	0	25	660	36	2	13	2 1/2 starch, 1 medium-fat meat, 3 fat
Tuscan Six Cheese	1 slice	410	23	5	8	0	25	760	37	1	15	2 1/2 starch, 1 medium-fat meat, 3 fat
The Works	1 slice	420	21	5	9	0	25	860	38	2	14	2 1/2 starch, 1 medium-fat meat, 3 1/2 fat

14" ORIGINAL CRUST PIZZAS

BBQ Chicken & Bacon Pizza	1 slice	340	11	3	3.5	0	30	960	44	2	15	3 starch, 1 medium-fat meat, 1 fat
Cheese	1 slice	300	11	3	3.5	0	20	750	39	2	13	2 1/2 starch, 1 medium-fat meat, 1 1/2 fat
Chicken Bacon Ranch	1 slice	340	14	4	3.5	0	25	700	38	2	15	2 1/2 starch, 1 medium-fat meat, 1 1/2 fat
Garden Fresh	1 slice	280	9	3	2.5	0	15	680	39	2	11	2 1/2 starch, 2 fat
Hawaiian BBQ Chicken	1 slice	340	11	3	3.5	0	30	960	46	2	16	3 starch, 1 medium-fat meat, 1 fat
Italian Meats Trio	1 slice	340	11	3	7	0	30	1030	38	2	16	2 1/2 starch, 1 medium-fat meat, 1 fat
The Meats	1 slice	350	16	4	5	0	30	930	38	2	15	2 1/2 starch, 1 medium-fat meat, 2 fat

(Continued)

✓ = Healthiest Bets

14" ORIGINAL CRUST PIZZAS *(Continued)*	Amount	Cal.	Fat (g)	% Cal. Fat	Sat. Fat (g)	Trans Fat (g)	Chol. (mg)	Sod. (mg)	Carb. (g)	Fiber (g)	Pro. (g)	Choices/Exchanges
Papa's White	1 slice	280	10	3	3.5	0	20	720	37	1	12	2 1/2 starch, 1 medium-fat meat, 1 fat
Pepperoni	1 slice	310	13	4	4	0	20	810	38	2	13	2 1/2 starch, 1 medium-fat meat, 2 fat
Sausage	1 slice	330	15	4	4.5	0	20	810	37	3	13	2 1/2 starch, 1 medium-fat meat, 2 fat
Sicilian Classic Pizza	1 slice	360	13	3	7	0	35	1060	38	3	16	2 1/2 starch, 1 medium-fat meat, 1 1/2 fat
Smokehouse Bacon & Ham	1 slice	330	13	4	3.5	0	30	890	39	2	16	2 1/2 starch, 1 medium-fat meat, 1 fat
Spicy Italian	1 slice	370	11	3	10	0	30	960	38	4	15	2 1/2 starch, 1 medium-fat meat, 1 fat
Spinach Alfredo	1 slice	280	11	4	4.5	0	20	630	36	2	11	2 1/2 starch, 1 medium-fat meat, 1 fat

Spinach Alfredo Chicken Tomato	1 slice	300	11	3	4.5	0	25	700	37	2	14	2 1/2 starch, 1 medium-fat meat, 1 fat
Tuscan Six Cheese	1 slice	320	13	4	4.5	0	25	780	38	2	15	2 1/2 starch, 1 medium-fat meat, 1 fat
The Works	1 slice	330	11	3	6	0	25	890	39	3	14	2 1/2 starch, 1 medium-fat meat, 1 1/2 fat

14" THIN CRUST PIZZAS

BBQ Chicken & Bacon Pizza	1 slice	290	14	4	3.5	0	30	740	29	<1	13	2 starch, 1 medium-fat meat, 2 fat
Cheese	1 slice	240	13	5	3.5	0	20	500	22	1	10	1 1/2 starch, 1 medium-fat meat, 2 fat
Chicken Bacon Ranch	1 slice	270	16	5	4	0	25	490	21	1	12	1 1/2 starch, 1 medium-fat meat, 2 fat
✔Garden Fresh	1 slice	210	11	5	2.5	0	15	430	23	2	8	1 1/2 starch, 2 fat
Hawaiian BBQ Chicken	1 slice	290	14	4	3.5	0	30	740	31	1	13	2 starch, 1 medium-fat meat, 2 fat

✔ = Healthiest Bets

(Continued)

14" THIN CRUST PIZZAS *(Continued)*	Amount	Cal.	Fat (g)	% Cal. Fat	Sat. Fat (g)	Trans Fat (g)	Chol. (mg)	Sod. (mg)	Carb. (g)	Fiber (g)	Pro. (g)	Choices/Exchanges
Italian Meats Trio	1 slice	280	12	4	7	0	30	820	22	2	13	1 1/2 starch, 1 medium-fat meat, 1 1/2 fat
The Meats	1 slice	300	18	5	5	0	30	700	23	2	13	1 1/2 starch, 1 medium-fat meat, 2 fat
Papa's White	1 slice	220	12	5	4	0	20	510	20	1	9	1 1/2 starch, 1 medium-fat meat, 1 1/2 fat
Pepperoni	1 slice	260	15	5	4.5	0	20	580	23	1	10	1 1/2 starch, 1 medium-fat meat, 2 fat
Sausage	1 slice	280	17	5	5	0	20	590	22	2	10	1 1/2 starch, 1 medium-fat meat, 2 1/2 fat
Sicilian Classic Pizza	1 slice	290	14	4	8	0	35	850	21	2	13	1 1/2 starch, 1 medium-fat meat, 2 fat
Smokehouse Bacon & Ham	1 slice	260	14	5	4	0	30	680	22	1	12	1 1/2 starch, 1 medium-fat meat, 1 1/2 fat

	Amount										Exchanges
Spicy Italian	1 slice	320	14	4	11	0	30	740	24	3	12	1 1/2 starch, 1 medium-fat meat, 2 fat
Spinach Alfredo	1 slice	220	13	5	4.5	0	20	370	19	1	8	1 1/2 starch, 1 medium-fat meat, 2 fat
Spinach Alfredo Chicken Tomato	1 slice	230	13	5	4.5	0	25	430	21	1	10	1 1/2 starch, 1 medium-fat meat, 2 fat
Tuscan Six Cheese	1 slice	250	14	5	5	0	25	570	21	1	12	1 1/2 starch, 1 medium-fat meat, 1 fat
The Works	1 slice	280	14	5	6	0	25	670	24	2	12	1 1/2 starch, 1 medium-fat meat, 2 fat

16" ORIGINAL CRUST PIZZAS

	Amount										Exchanges
BBQ Chicken & Bacon Pizza	1 slice	370	13	3	4	0	30	1050	48	2	17	3 starch, 1 medium-fat meat, 1 fat
Cheese	1 slice	310	11	3	3.5	0	20	760	41	2	13	2 1/2 starch, 1 medium-fat meat, 1 fat

(Continued)

✔ = Healthiest Bets

16" ORIGINAL CRUST PIZZAS *(Continued)*	Amount	Cal.	Fat (g)	% Cal. Fat	Sat. Fat (g)	Trans Fat (g)	Chol. (mg)	Sod. (mg)	Carb. (g)	Fiber (g)	Pro. (g)	Choices/Exchanges
Chicken Bacon Ranch	1 slice	370	16	4	4.5	0	30	790	41	2	17	2 1/2 starch, 1 medium-fat meat, 2 fat
Garden Fresh	1 slice	310	10	3	3	0	15	760	43	2	13	3 starch, 1 medium-fat meat, 1 fat
Hawaiian BBQ Chicken	1 slice	370	13	3	4	0	30	1010	48	2	17	3 starch, 1 medium-fat meat, 1 fat
Italian Meats Trio	1 slice	380	12	3	8	0	35	1160	41	3	18	2 1/2 starch, 1 medium-fat meat, 1 1/2 fat
The Meats	1 slice	390	18	4	6	0	35	1040	41	2	17	2 1/2 starch, 1 medium-fat meat, 2 fat
Papa's White	1 slice	310	12	3	4	0	25	810	40	1	13	2 1/2 starch, 1 medium-fat meat, 1 fat
Pepperoni	1 slice	350	15	4	5	0	25	910	41	2	15	2 1/2 starch, 1 medium-fat meat, 2 fat

Sausage	1 slice	370	18	4	5	0	25	910	41	3	14	2 1/2 starch, 1 medium-fat meat, 3 fat
Sicilian Classic Pizza	1 slice	400	15	3	8	0	40	1190	41	3	18	2 1/2 starch, 1 medium-fat meat, 1 1/2 fat
Smokehouse Bacon & Ham	1 slice	370	15	4	4.5	0	35	1010	42	2	18	3 starch, 1 medium-fat meat, 1 fat
Spicy Italian	1 slice	410	13	3	11	0	35	1070	42	4	17	3 starch, 1 medium-fat meat, 2 fat
Spinach Alfredo	1 slice	320	13	4	5	0	25	710	39	2	13	2 1/2 starch, 1 medium-fat meat, 2 fat
Spinach Alfredo Chicken Tomato	1 slice	340	13	3	5	0	30	790	41	2	16	2 1/2 starch, 1 medium-fat meat, 1 1/2 fat
Tuscan Six Cheese	1 slice	340	13	3	5	0	25	820	41	2	16	2 1/2 starch, 1 medium-fat meat, 1 1/2 fat
The Works	1 slice	370	13	3	7	0	30	1000	42	3	16	3 starch, 1 medium-fat meat, 1 1/2 fat

(Continued)

✔ = Healthiest Bets

	Amount	Cal.	Fat (g)	% Cal. Fat	Sat. Fat (g)	Trans Fat (g)	Chol. (mg)	Sod. (mg)	Carb. (g)	Fiber (g)	Pro. (g)	Choices/Exchanges
BREADSTICKS												
Garlic Parmesan	2 sticks	330	10	3	1.5	0	0	720	54	2	10	3 1/2 starch, 2 fat
Plain	2 sticks	290	5	2	0.5	0	0	540	53	2	9	3 1/2 starch, 1 fat
Whole Wheat	2 sticks	270	5	2	0.5	0	0	500	53	8	8	3 1/2 starch, 1 fat
DESSERTS												
Apple Twist Sweetreat	2 slices	380	16	4	4	0	0	530	54	1	5	3 1/2 carb, 2 fat
Chocolate Pastry Delights	1 pastry	180	11	6	6	0	5	140	18	1	2	1 carb, 2 fat
Cinna Swirl Sweetreat	2 slices	420	21	5	5	0	0	570	53	1	5	3 1/2 carb, 3 fat
Cinnamon Sweetsticks	4 sticks	570	15	2	3	0	0	750	98	3	12	6 1/2 carb, 2 fat
DIPPING SAUCES												
✓Barbeque Sauce	1 cup	40	0	0	0	0	0	240	11	0	0	1/2 carb
Blue Cheese	1 cup	170	18	10	3.5	0	20	240	1	0	1	3 1/2 fat

	Serving Size	Cal.	Fat (g)	% Fat Cal.	Sat. Fat (g)	Chol. (mg)	Sod. (mg)	Carb. (g)	Fiber (g)	Prot. (g)	Exchanges
Buffalo Sauce	1 cup	15	0.5	30	0	0	890	2	0	0	Free
Cheese Sauce	1 cup	70	6	8	1.5	0	150	1	0	1	1 1/2 fat
Honey Mustard	1 cup	150	15	9	2	10	120	5	0	0	1/2 carb, 3 fat
✔ Pizza Sauce	1 cup	20	0	0	0	0	140	3	0	0	Free
Ranch Sauce	1 cup	110	11	9	2	10	250	1	0	1	2 fat
Special Garlic	1 cup	150	17	10	3	0	310	0	0	0	3 1/2 fat
SEASONINGS											
✔ Crushed Red Pepper	1 pkt	5	0	0	0	n/a	n/a	0	1	0	Free
✔ Parmesan Cheese	1 pkt	15	1	6	0.5	n/a	5	45	0	0	Free
✔ Special Seasonings	1 pkt	5	0	0	0	n/a	0	410	1	0	Free
SIDES											
BBQ Wings	2 wings	200	12	5	3.5	105	700	6	0	17	1/2 starch, 2 lean meat, 1 fat

✔ = Healthiest Bets

(Continued)

218 *Papa John's Pizza*

SIDES *(Continued)*	Amount	Cal.	Fat (g)	% Cal. Fat	Sat. Fat (g)	Trans Fat (g)	Chol. (mg)	Sod. (mg)	Carb. (g)	Fiber (g)	Pro. (g)	Choices/Exchanges
Buffalo Wings	2 wings	200	14	6	4	0	110	840	1	1	18	3 lean meat, 1 1/2 fat
Cheesesticks	4 sticks	370	16	4	4.5	0	25	830	42	2	15	3 starch, 1 medium-fat meat, 2 fat
Chickenstrips	2 strips	160	8	5	2	0	25	350	10	0	10	1/2 starch, 1 lean meat, 1 fat

✔ = Healthiest Bets

Pizza Hut
(www.pizzahut.com)

Light 'n Lean Choice

12" Fit 'N' Delicious Pizza, Diced Chicken, Mushroom, and Jalapeño (3 slices)

Calories......................480
Fat (g) 15
   % calories from fat..28
   Saturated fat (g) 6
   Trans fat (g) 0

Cholesterol (mg) 45
Sodium (mg) 2,190
Carbohydrate (g).........66
   Fiber (g).....................3
Protein (g) 27

Exchanges: 4 1/2 starch, 1 veg, 2 medium-fat meat

Healthy 'n Hearty Choice

14" Fit 'N' Delicious Pizza, Ham, Pineapple, and Diced Red Tomato (3 slices)

Calories......................690
Fat (g) 18
   % calories from fat..23
   Saturated fat (g) 7.5
   Trans fat (g) 0

Cholesterol (mg) 60
Sodium (mg) 2,490
Carbohydrate (g).........96
   Fiber (g).....................3
Protein (g) 33

Exchanges: 6 1/2 starch, 1 veg, 2 medium-fat meat, 1 1/2 fat

Pizza Hut

12" FIT N' DELICIOUS PIZZA

	Amount	Cal.	Fat (g)	% Cal. Fat	Sat. Fat (g)	Trans Fat (g)	Chol. (mg)	Sod. (mg)	Carb. (g)	Fiber (g)	Pro. (g)	Choices/Exchanges
Diced Chicken, Mushroom, & Jalapeno	1 slice	160	5	3	2	0	15	730	22	1	9	1 1/2 starch, 1 medium-fat meat
Diced Chicken, Red Onion & Green Pepper	1 slice	170	5	3	2	0	15	520	23	1	9	1 1/2 starch, 1 medium-fat meat, 1/2 fat
Diced Red Tomato, Mushroom & Jalapeno	1 slice	150	4	2	1.5	0	10	630	22	1	6	1 1/2 starch, 1 fat
✓Green Pepper, & Diced Red Tomato	1 slice	150	4	2	1.5	0	10	420	23	1	6	1 1/2 starch, 1 medium-fat meat
Ham, Pineapple, & Diced Red Tomato	1 slice	160	5	3	2	0	15	580	13	1	8	1 starch, 1 medium-fat meat, 1 fat

											Exchanges/Choices
Ham, Red Onion, & Mushroom	1 slice	160	5	3	2	0	15	580	23	1	8	1 1/2 starch, 1 medium-fat meat

12" MEDIUM HAND-TOSSED STYLE PIZZA

											Exchanges/Choices
Cheese Only	1 slice	230	10	4	4.5	1	25	620	25	1	12	1 1/2 starch, 1 medium-fat meat, 1 fat
Italian Sausage & Red Onion	1 slice	260	12	4	5	1	30	670	26	1	12	1 1/2 starch, 1 medium-fat meat, 1 1/2 fat
Meat Lovers	1 slice	340	19	5	7	1	45	1040	25	1	17	1 1/2 starch, 2 medium-fat meat, 2 fat
Pepperoni	1 slice	240	11	4	4.5	1	25	690	24	1	12	1 1/2 starch, 1 medium-fat meat, 1 fat
Pepperoni & Mushroom	1 slice	230	9	4	4	1	20	610	25	1	11	1 1/2 starch, 1 medium-fat meat, 1 fat
Quartered Ham & Pineapple	1 slice	220	8	3	3.5	1	20	620	26	1	10	1 1/2 starch, 1 medium-fat meat, 1 fat

(Continued)

✓ = Healthiest Bets

12" MEDIUM HAND-TOSSED STYLE PIZZA *(Continued)*	Amount	Cal.	Fat (g)	% Cal. Fat	Sat. Fat (g)	Trans Fat (g)	Chol. (mg)	Sod. (mg)	Carb. (g)	Fiber (g)	Pro. (g)	Choices/Exchanges
Supreme	1 slice	270	13	4	5	1	30	780	26	2	13	1 1/2 starch, 1 medium-fat meat, 1 fat
Veggie Lovers	1 slice	210	8	3	3.5	1	15	580	26	2	10	1 1/2 starch, 1 medium-fat meat, 1 fat
12" MEDIUM PAN PIZZA												
Cheese Only	1 slice	270	13	4	5	0	25	570	27	1	11	2 starch, 1 medium-fat meat, 2 fat
Italian Sausage & Red Onion	1 slice	300	15	5	5	0	30	610	38	1	12	2 1/2 starch, 1 medium-fat meat, 2 fat
Meat Lovers	1 slice	370	22	5	8	0	45	990	28	2	17	2 starch, 2 medium-fat meat, 3 fat
Pepperoni	1 slice	260	14	5	5	0	25	640	27	1	12	2 starch, 1 medium-fat meat, 2 fat
Pepperoni & Mushroom	1 slice	260	13	5	4.85	0	20	560	27	1	11	2 starch, 1 medium-fat meat, 2 fat

Quartered Ham & Pineapple	1 slice	250	11	4	4	0	20	560	28	1	10
Supreme	1 slice	310	16	5	6	0	30	720	28	2	13
Veggie Lovers	1 slice	250	11	4	4	0	15	530	28	2	10

12" MEDIUM THIN N' CRISPY PIZZA

Cheese Only	1 slice	200	8	4	4.5	0	25	570	21	1	10
Italian Sausage & Red Onion	1 slice	230	11	4	4.5	0	30	620	23	1	10
Meat Lovers	1 slice	310	18	5	7	0.5	45	1010	22	1	15
Pepperoni	1 slice	210	10	4	4.5	0	25	640	21	1	10

Exchanges:
- Quartered Ham & Pineapple: 2 starch, 1 medium-fat meat, 1 1/2 fat
- Supreme: 2 starch, 1 medium-fat meat, 2 fat
- Veggie Lovers: 2 starch, 1 medium-fat meat, 1 1/2 fat
- Cheese Only: 1 1/2 starch, 1 medium-fat meat, 1 fat
- Italian Sausage & Red Onion: 1 1/2 starch, 1 medium-fat meat, 1 1/2 fat
- Meat Lovers: 1 1/2 starch, 2 medium-fat meat, 2 fat
- Pepperoni: 1 1/2 starch, 1 medium-fat meat, 1 fat

(Continued)

✓ = Healthiest Bets

12" MEDIUM THIN N' CRISPY PIZZA (Continued)

	Amount	Cal.	Cal. Fat	Fat (g)	% Fat Fat	Sat. Fat (g)	Trans Fat (g)	Chol. (mg)	Sod. (mg)	Carb. (g)	Fiber (g)	Pro. (g)	Choices/Exchanges
Pepperoni & Mushroom	1 slice	190		8	4	3.5	0	20	560	21	1	9	1 1/2 starch, 1 medium-fat meat, 1 fat
Quartered Ham & Pineapple	1 slice	180		6	3	3	0	20	570	23	1	9	1 1/2 starch, 1 medium-fat meat, 1/2 fat
Supreme	1 slice	230		11	4	5	0	30	730	22	1	11	1 1/2 starch, 1 medium-fat meat, 1 1/2 fat
Veggie Lovers	1 slice	180		7	4	3	0	15	550	23	1	8	1 1/2 starch, 1 1/2 fat
14" LARGE HAND-TOSSED STYLE PIZZA													
Cheese Only	1 slice	340		14	4	7	1.5	35	900	36	2	17	2 1/2 starch, 1 medium-fat meat, 1 fat
Italian Sausage & Red Onion	1 slice	370		17	4	7	1.5	40	960	38	2	17	2 1/2 starch, 1 medium-fat meat, 2 fat
Meat Lovers	1 slice	490		27	5	11	1.5	65	1510	37	2	24	2 1/2 starch, 2 medium-fat meat, 3 fat

Pepperoni	1 slice	380	15	4	7	1.5	40	1010	35	2	17	2 1/2 starch, 1 medium-fat meat, 2 fat
Pepperoni & Mushroom	1 slice	330	14	4	6	1.5	30	890	36	2	16	2 1/2 starch, 1 medium-fat meat, 1 fat
Quartered Ham & Pineapple	1 slice	310	11	3	5	1.5	30	900	38	2	15	2 1/2 starch, 1 medium-fat meat, 1 fat
Supreme	1 slice	390	18	4	8	1.5	40	1130	37	2	19	2 1/2 starch, 2 medium-fat meat, 2 fat
Veggie Lovers	1 slice	310	12	3	5	1.5	25	840	37	2	14	2 1/2 starch, 1 medium-fat meat, 1 fat

14" FIT N' DELICIOUS PIZZA

Diced Chicken, Mushroom, & Jalapeno	1 slice	230	6	2	2.5	0	25	1010	43	2	13	3 starch, 1 medium-fat meat
Diced Chicken, Red Onion & Green Pepper	1 slice	230	8	3	2.5	0	25	730	32	2	13	2 starch, 1 medium-fat meat

(Continued)

✔ = Healthiest Bets

14" FIT N' DELICIOUS PIZZA (Continued)	Amount	Cal.	Fat (g)	% Cal. Fat	Sat. Fat (g)	Trans Fat (g)	Chol. (mg)	Sod. (mg)	Carb. (g)	Fiber (g)	Pro. (g)	Choices/Exchanges
Diced Red Tomato, Mushroom & Jalapeno	1 slice	210	6	3	2.5	0	10	870	31	2	9	2 starch, 1 fat
Green Pepper, & Diced Red Tomato	1 slice	210	6	3	2.5	0	10	580	32	2	8	2 starch, 1 fat
Ham, Pineapple, & Diced Red Tomato	1 slice	230	6	2	2.5	0	20	830	32	1	11	2 starch, 1 medium-fat meat, 1/2 fat
Ham, Red Onion, & Mushroom	1 slice	230	7	3	205	0	20	820	31	2	11	2 starch, 1 medium-fat meat, 1/2 fat
14" LARGE PAN PIZZA												
Cheese Only	1 slice	390	19	4	7	0	35	800	38	2	18	2 1/2 starch, 1 medium-fat meat, 2 fat
Italian Sausage & Red Onion	1 slice	420	22	5	8	0	40	860	39	2	17	2 1/2 starch, 1 medium-fat meat, 3 fat
Meat Lovers	1 slice	530	31	5	11	0.5	65	1400	39	2	23	2 1/2 starch, 2 medium-fat meat, 4 fat

	Amount										Servings/Exchanges
Pepperoni	1 slice	400	21	5	7	0	40	900	37	2	18	2 1/2 starch, 2 medium-fat meat, 2 fat
Pepperoni & Mushroom	1 slice	380	18	4	6	0	30	790	37	2	15	2 1/2 starch, 1 medium-fat meat, 2 1/2 fat
Quartered Ham & Pineapple	1 slice	360	16	4	6	0	30	790	39	2	15	2 1/2 starch, 1 medium-fat meat, 2 fat
Supreme	1 slice	440	23	5	7	0.5	40	1020	30	2	18	2 starch, 2 medium-fat meat, 3 fat
Veggie Lovers	1 slice	350	16	4	6	0	25	730	39	2	14	2 1/2 starch, 1 medium-fat meat, 2 fat

14" LARGE STUFFED CRUST PIZZA

	Amount										Servings/Exchanges
Cheese Only	1 slice	360	16	4	5	1.5	40	1050	37	2	18	2 1/2 starch, 2 medium-fat meat, 1 fat
Italian Sausage & Red Onion	1 slice	410	20	4	9	1.5	50	1190	39	2	19	2 1/2 starch, 2 medium-fat meat, 2 fat

(Continued)

✔ = Healthiest Bets

14" LARGE STUFFED CRUST PIZZA (Continued)	Amount	Cal.	Fat (g)	% Cal. Fat	Sat. Fat (g)	Trans Fat (g)	Chol. (mg)	Sod. (mg)	Carb. (g)	Fiber (g)	Pro. (g)	Choices/Exchanges
Meat Lovers	1 slice	620	29	4	12	2	75	1690	39	2	26	2 1/2 starch, 3 medium-fat meat, 5 fat
Pepperoni	1 slice	390	16	4	7	1.5	50	1320	39	2	19	2 1/2 starch, 2 medium-fat meat, 1 1/2 fat
Pepperoni & Mushroom	1 slice	360	18	5	7	1.5	40	1090	37	2	18	2 1/2 starch, 2 medium-fat meat, 2 fat
Quartered Ham & Pineapple	1 slice	350	14	4	7	1.5	40	1090	39	2	17	2 1/2 starch, 1 medium-fat meat, 1 fat
Supreme	1 slice	420	21	5	9	1.5	50	1320	39	2	21	2 1/2 starch, 2 medium-fat meat, 2 fat
Veggie Lovers	1 slice	340	14	4	7	1.5	35	1030	38	2	16	2 1/2 starch, 1 medium-fat meat, 1 fat

14" LARGE THIN N' CRISPY PIZZA

Cheese Only	1 slice	280	12	4	6	0	35	810	30	1	14	2 starch, 1 medium-fat meat, 1 fat
Italian Sausage & Red Onion	1 slice	320	15	4	7	0	40	870	32	2	14	2 starch, 1 medium-fat meat, 2 fat
Meat Lovers	1 slice	430	25	5	10	0.5	65	1430	31	2	21	2 starch, 2 medium-fat meat, 3 fat
Pepperoni	1 slice	300	14	4	6	0	40	920	29	1	14	2 starch, 1 medium-fat meat, 1 1/2 fat
Pepperoni & Mushroom	1 slice	270	12	4	5	0	30	800	30	1	13	2 starch, 1 medium-fat meat, 1 fat
Quartered Ham & Pineapple	1 slice	260	9	3	4.5	0	30	810	32	1	12	2 starch, 1 medium-fat meat, 1 fat
Supreme	1 slice	330	16	4	7	0.5	40	1040	31	2	16	2 starch, 1 medium-fat meat, 2 fat

✔ = Healthiest Bets

(Continued)

14" LARGE THIN N' CRISPY PIZZA (*Continued*)	Amount	Cal.	Fat (g)	% Cal. Fat	Sat. Fat (g)	Trans Fat (g)	Chol. (mg)	Sod. (mg)	Carb. (g)	Fiber (g)	Pro. (g)	Choices/Exchanges
Veggie Lovers	1 slice	260	10	3	4.5	0	25	770	31	2	12	2 starch, 1 medium-fat meat, 1 fat
6" PERSONAL PAN PIZZA												
Cheese Only	Whole Pizza	620	26	4	11	0.5	60	1370	69	3	28	4 1/2 starch, 2 medium-fat meat, 2 fat
Italian Sausage & Red Onion	Whole Pizza	690	33	4	12	0.5	70	1530	71	4	29	4 1/2 starch, 2 medium-fat meat, 4 fat
Meat Lovers	Whole Pizza	890	49	5	18	1	115	2460	70	4	41	4 1/2 starch, 4 medium-fat meat, 5 fat
Pepperoni	Whole Pizza	640	29	4	11	0.5	65	1530	67	3	28	4 1/2 starch, 2 medium-fat meat, 3 fat
Pepperoni & Mushroom	Whole Pizza	600	25	4	10	0.5	55	1350	68	3	26	4 1/2 starch, 2 medium-fat meat, 2 1/2 fat

Quartered Ham & Pineapple	Whole Pizza	570	21	3	8	0	50	1380	70	3	25	4 1/2 starch, 2 medium-fat meat, 2 fat
Supreme	Whole Pizza	710	34	4	13	1	70	1800	70	4	32	4 1/2 starch, 3 medium-fat meat, 3 fat
Veggie Lovers	Whole Pizza	560	22	4	8	0	40	1250	70	4	24	4 1/2 starch, 1 medium-fat meat, 2 fat

APPETIZERS

✔ Breadsticks	1	150	6	4	1	0	0	230	20	1	4	1 1/2 starch, 1 fat
Cheese Breadsticks	1	200	10	5	3	0	15	370	21	1	7	1 1/2 starch, 2 fat
Hot Wings	2 pcs	120	7	5	2	0	65	500	1	0	11	2 lean meat, 1/2 fat
Mild Wings	2 pcs	110	7	6	2	0	65	390	2	0	11	2 lean meat, 1/2 fat

DESSERTS

Apple Dessert Pizza	1 slice	260	5	2	1	0.5	0	290	52	1	4	3 1/2 carb, 1/2 fat
Cherry Dessert Pizza	1 slice	260	4.5	2	1	0.5	0	280	47	1	4	3 carb, 1 fat

✔ = Healthiest Bets

(Continued)

DESSERTS (Continued)	Amount	Cal.	Fat (g)	% Cal. Fat	Sat. Fat (g)	Trans Fat (g)	Chol. (mg)	Sod. (mg)	Carb. (g)	Fiber (g)	Pro. (g)	Choices/Exchanges
✓Cinnamon Sticks	2 pcs	170	5	3	1	0	0	180	27	1	4	2 carb, 1 fat
White Icing Dipping Cup	2 oz.	190	0	0	0	0	0	0	47	0	0	3 carb
DIPPING SAUCES												
✓Breadstick	3 oz.	40	0	0	0	0	0	270	8	0	1	1/2 carb
Wing Blue Cheese	1.5 oz.	220	23	9	4	0	15	400	3	0	1	4 1/2 fat
Wing Ranch	1.5 oz.	220	23	9	4	0	25	400	3	0	1	4 1/2 fat
DRESSINGS												
French	2 Tbsp.	150	13	8	2	0	0	180	9	0	0	1/2 carb, 2 1/2 fat
Italian	2 Tbsp.	140	15	10	2.5	0	0	360	2	0	0	3 fat
✓Lite Italian	2 Tbsp.	70	5	6	1	0	0	510	5	0	0	1/2 carb, 1 fat
✓Lite Ranch	2 Tbsp.	60	6	9	1	0	15	260	1	0	0	1 fat
✓Ranch	2 Tbsp.	100	10	9	1.5	0	5	220	2	0	1	2 fat

Thousand Island	2 Tbsp.	120	11	8	1.5	0	10	220	5	0	0	1/2 carb, 2 fat

XL FULL HOUSE PIZZA

Cheese Only	1 slice	260	12	4	5	0	30	690	30	2	12	2 starch, 1 medium-fat meat, 1 fat
Italian Sausage & Red Onion	1 slice	300	14	4	5	0	30	720	32	2	12	2 starch, 1 medium-fat meat, 2 fat
Meat Lovers	1 slice	370	20	5	8	0	45	1090	31	2	17	2 starch, 2 medium-fat meat, 2 fat
Pepperoni	1 slice	280	13	4	5	0	30	750	30	2	12	2 starch, 1 medium-fat meat, 1 1/2 fat
Pepperoni & Mushroom	1 slice	270	11	4	1.5	0	25	670	30	2	11	2 starch, 1 medium-fat meat, 1 1/2 fat
Quartered Ham & Pineapple	1 slice	260	10	3	4	0	20	680	32	2	11	2 starch, 1 medium-fat meat, 1 fat

✔ = Healthiest Bets

(Continued)

XL FULL HOUSE PIZZA (*Continued*)	Amount	Cal.	Fat (g)	% Cal. Fat	Sat. Fat (g)	Trans Fat (g)	Chol. (mg)	Sod. (mg)	Carb. (g)	Fiber (g)	Pro. (g)	Choices/Exchanges
Supreme	1 slice	310	14	4	6	0	30	830	31	2	13	2 starch, 1 medium-fat meat, 2 fat
Veggie Lovers	1 slice	260	10	3	4	0	20	650	31	2	10	2 starch, 1 medium-fat meat, 1 1/2 fat

✔ = Healthiest Bets

Starbucks (www.starbucks.com)

Light 'n Lean Choice

Raspberry Scone (1/2)
Caffe Latte, non-fat (12 oz)

Calories	345	Cholesterol (mg)	48
Fat (g)	11	Sodium (mg)	400
% calories from fat	29	Carbohydrate (g)	48
Saturated fat (g)	6	Fiber (g)	1
Trans fat (g)	0	Protein (g)	14

Exchanges: 2 carb, 1 fat-free milk, 2 fat

Healthy 'n Hearty Choice

Cranberry Orange Muffin
Coffee Frappuccino, with nonfat milk (12 oz)

Calories	520	Cholesterol (mg)	85
Fat (g)	12	Sodium (mg)	730
% calories from fat	21	Carbohydrate (g)	98
Saturated fat (g)	6.5	Fiber (g)	2
Trans fat (g)	0	Protein (g)	9

Exchanges: 5 1/2 carb, 1 milk, 2 1/2 fat

Starbucks

BROWNIES, COOKIES, & BARS

	Amount	Cal.	Fat (g)	% Cal. Fat	Sat. Fat (g)	Trans Fat (g)	Chol. (mg)	Sod. (mg)	Carb. (g)	Fiber (g)	Pro. (g)	Choices/Exchanges
Black and White Cookie	1	240	12	5	1	0	40	160	32	1	2	2 carb, 2 1/2 fat
Blueberry Oat Bar w/ Organic Blueberries	1	390	15	3	5	0	0	300	59	3		4 carb, 5 medium-fat meat, 3 fat
Chewy Marshmallow Square	1	280	6	2	3	0	10	330	54	0	2	3 1/2 carb, 1 fat
Chocolate Chunk Cookie	1	370	18	4	11	0	60	150	50	2	4	3 1/2 carb, 3 1/2 fat
Chocolate Fudge Brownie	1	410	22	5	13	0	110	136	52	2	5	3 1/2 carb, 4 1/2 fat
Decorated Cookie	1	470	14	3	8	0	60	130	80	1	5	5 carb, 3 fat
Lemon Slice Cookie	1	460	22	4	10	0	25	250	60	1	5	4 carb, 4 fat
Oatmeal Raisin Cookie	1	350	12	3	7	0	50	95	56	3	5	3 1/2 carb, 2 1/2 fat

Rainbow Cookie	1	480	20	4	13	1	70	210	71	1	6	4 1/2 carb, 4 fat
Toffee Almond Bar	1	400	19	4	8	0	50	340	53	1	4	3 1/2 carb, 4 fat

CLASSIC FAVORITES - NONFAT

Apple Juice	12 oz	190	0	0	0	0	0	20	48	0	0	3 carb
Caramel Apple Spice - no whip	12 oz	240	0	0	0	0	0	20	57	0	0	4 carb
Caramel Apple Spice - whip	12 oz	300	7	2	4	0	25	25	59	0	0	4 carb
Chocolate Milk	12 oz	220	2	1	0	0	5	150	41	1	14	1 1/2 carb, 1 1/2 milk
Cinnamon Dolce Crème - no whip	12 oz	170	0	0	0	0	5	120	31	0	10	2 carb
Cinnamon Dolce Crème - whip	12 oz	230	6	2	4	0	30	25	33	0	10	2 carb, 1 fat
✔ Honey Crème - no whip	12 oz	160	0	0	0	0	5	125	29	0	10	2 carb

(Continued)

✔ = Healthiest Bets

CLASSIC FAVORITES -, NONFAT *(Continued)*	Amount	Cal.	Fat (g)	% Cal. Fat	Sat. Fat (g)	Trans Fat (g)	Chol. (mg)	Sod. (mg)	Carb. (g)	Fiber (g)	Pro. (g)	Choices/Exchanges
Honey Crème - whip	12 oz	230	6	2	4	0	30	130	33	0	10	2 carb, 1 fat
Hot Chocolate - no whip	12 oz	190	2	1	0	0	5	110	37	1	11	1 1/2 carb, 1 milk
Hot Chocolate - whip	12 oz	250	8	3	4	0	30	115	39	1	11	2 carb, 1 milk, 1 1/2 fat
Pumpkin Spice Crème - no whip	12 oz	200	0	0	0	0	25	180	39	0	12	2 1/2 carb, 1 milk
Pumpkin Spice Crème - whip	12 oz	260	6	2	4	0	30	180	40	0	12	3 carb, 1 milk, 1 fat
Steamed Apple Juice	12 oz	170	0	0	0	0	0	15	43	0	0	3 carb
✔Vanilla Crème - no whip	12 oz	150	0	0	0	0	5	120	28	0	10	2 carb
Vanilla Crème - whip	12 oz	220	6	2	4	0	30	125	30	0	10	2 carb, 1 fat
White Hot Chocolate - no whip	12 oz	270	5	2	3.5	0	5	200	47	0	12	1 carb, 11 1/2 milk, 1 fat

White Hot Chocolate - whip	12 oz	330	10	3	7	0	20	100	49	0	12	1 carb, 1 1/2 milk, 2 fat

CROISSANTS, BAGELS & BREADS

8 Grain Roll	1	270	1	0	0.5	0	0	400	56	5	8	3 1/2 starch
Butter Croissant	1	300	15	5	9	0	45	350	36	1	5	2 starch, 3 fat
Chocolate Croissant	1	470	26	5	13	0.5	60	440	65	2	7	4 starch, 5 fat
Plain Bagel	1	310	2	1	0.5	0	0	600	61	2	11	4 starch

DOUGHNUTS, SWEET ROLLS & DANISH

Artisan Cinnamon Roll	1	400	22	5	10	0	20	310	48	1	4	3 carb, 4 1/2 fat
Cheese Danish	1	390	19	4	12	0.5	50	410	47	2	8	3 carb, 4 fat
Cinnamon Twist	1	420	20	4	12	0.5	50	400	51	2	8	3 1/2 carb, 4 fat
Top Pot Apple Fritter	1	490	22	4	10	0	0	290	65	1	4	4 carb, 4 1/2 fat
Top Pot Chocolate Old Fashioned Doughnut	1	480	25	5	7	0	20	350	60	2	5	4 carb, 5 fat

✔ = Healthiest Bets

(Continued)

DOUGHNUTS, SWEET ROLLS-, & DANISH *(Continued)*	Amount	Cal.	Fat (g)	% Cal. Fat	Sat. Fat (g)	Trans Fat (g)	Chol. (mg)	Sod. (mg)	Carb. (g)	Fiber (g)	Pro. (g)	Choices/Exchanges
✓Top Pot Glazed Old Fashioned Mini Doughnut	1	150	7	4	1.5	0	5	120	19	0	1	1 carb, 1 1/2 fat

FRAPPUCCINO BLENDED COFFEE - NONFAT MILK

	Amount	Cal.	Fat (g)	% Cal. Fat	Sat. Fat (g)	Trans Fat (g)	Chol. (mg)	Sod. (mg)	Carb. (g)	Fiber (g)	Pro. (g)	Choices/Exchanges
Caffe Vanilla - no whip	12 oz	230	3	1	1.5	0	10	180	49	0	4	2 1/2 carb, 1 milk, 1/2 fat
Caffe Vanilla - whip	12 oz	320	10	3	6	0	40	190	52	0	4	2 1/2 carb, 1 milk, 2 fat
Caramel - no whip	12 oz	220	3	1	2	0	10	180	44	0	4	2 carb, 1 milk, 1/2 fat
Caramel - whip	12 oz	300	11	3	7	0	40	190	46	0	4	2 carb, 1 milk, 2 fat
Cinnamon Dolce - no whip	12 oz	210	3	1	1.5	0	10	180	43	0	4	2 carb, 1 milk, 1/2 fat
Cinnamon Dolce - whip	12 oz	290	10	3	6	0	40	190	45	0	4	2 carb, 1 milk, 2 fat
Espresso	12 oz	180	3	2	1.5	0	10	170	37	0	4	1 1/2 carb, 1 milk, 1/2 fat
Honey - no whip	12 oz	210	3	1	1.5	0	10	180	44	0	4	2 carb, 1 milk, 1/2 fat
Honey - whip	12 oz	300	10	3	6	0	40	180	47	0	4	2 carb, 1 milk, 2 fat

	Size											Exchanges
Java Chip - no whip	12 oz	260	6	2	4	0	10	480	50	1	5	2 1/2 carb, 1 milk, 1 fat
Java Chip - whip	12 oz	340	14	4	9	0	40	180	52	1	6	2 1/2 carb, 1 milk, 3 fat
Mint Mocha Chip - no whip	12 oz	270	5	2	3.5	0	10	200	54	1	5	3 carb, 1 milk, 1 fat
Mint Mocha Chip - whip	12 oz	360	14	4	9	0	40	210	57	1	6	3 carb, 1 milk, 3 fat
Mocha - no whip	12 oz	200	3	1	1.5	0	10	170	41	0	4	1 carb, 1 milk, 1/2 fat
Mocha - whip	12 oz	280	11	4	6	0	40	180	43	0	5	1 1/2 carb, 1 milk, 2 fat
Pumpkin Spice - no whip	12 oz	230	3	1	1.5	0	10	210	47	0	5	1 1/2 carb, 1 milk, 1/2 fat
Pumpkin Spice - whip	12 oz	310	11	3	7	0	40	210	49	0	5	2 carb, 1 milk, 2 fat
White Chocolate Mocha - no whip	12 oz	240	4	2	2.5	0	10	200	47	1	5	2 carb, 1 milk, 1 fat
White Chocolate Mocha - whip	12 oz	320	12	3	7	0	40	210	49	0	5	2 1/2 carb, 2 1/2 milk

(Continued)

✔ = Healthiest Bets

	Amount	Cal.	Fat (g)	% Cal. Fat	Sat. Fat (g)	Trans Fat (g)	Chol. (mg)	Sod. (mg)	Carb. (g)	Fiber (g)	Pro. (g)	Choices/Exchanges
FRAPPUCCINO BLENDED CRÈME - NONFAT												
Double Chocolaty Chip - no whip	12 oz	300	6	2	0	0	5	230	57	2	10	3 carb, 1 milk, 1 fat
Double Chocolaty Chip - whip	12 oz	380	14	3	8	0	35	240	59	2	11	3 carb, 1 milk, 3 fat
Honey - no whip	12 oz	250	2	1	0	0	5	240	50	1	8	2 1/2 carb, 1 milk
Honey - whip	12 oz	330	10	3	5	0	35	250	53	1	9	2 1/2 carb, 1 milk, 2 fat
Mint Chocolaty Chip - no whip	12 oz	310	5	1	2	0	5	240	61	2	9	3 carb, 1 milk, 1 fat
Mint Chocolaty Chip - whip	12 oz	400	14	3	8	0	35	250	64	2	10	3 carb, 1 milk, 3 fat
Pumpkin Spice - no whip	12 oz	280	2	1	0	0	5	270	55	0	10	3 carb, 1 milk
Pumpkin Spice - whip	12 oz	360	10	3	5	0	35	380	58	0	10	3 carb, 1 milk, 2 fat

Strawberries and Crème - no whip	12 oz	320	2	1	0	0	5	240	66	0	9	3 1/2 carb, 1 milk
Strawberries and Crème - whip	12 oz	410	11	2	6	0	40	250	68	0	9	3 1/2 carb, 1 milk, 2 fat
Tazo Chai - no whip	12 oz	260	2	1	0	0	5	220	52	0	8	2 1/2 carb, 1 milk
Tazo Chai - whip	12 oz	340	10	3	5	0	24	120	55	0	9	3 carb, 1 milk, 2 fat
Tazo Green Tea - no whip	12 oz	290	2	1	0	0	5	230	60	1	9	3 carb, 1 milk
Tazo Green Tea - whip	12 oz	370	10	2	5	0	35	240	62	1	9	3 carb, 1 milk, 2 fat
Vanilla Bean - no whip	12 oz	260	2	1	0	0	5	230	53	0	9	2 1/2 carb, 1 milk
Vanilla Bean - whip	12 oz	340	10	3	5	0	35	240	55	0	9	3 carb, 1 milk, 2 fat
FRAPPUCCINO LIGHT BLENDED COFFEE - NONFAT												
✔Caffe Vanilla	12 oz	140	1	1	0	0	0	180	30	2	4	2 carb
✔Caramel	12 oz	130	1	1	0	0	5	180	25	2	4	1 1/2 carb

(Continued)

✔ = Healthiest Bets

FRAPPUCCINO LIGHT BLENDED COFFEE - NONFAT *(Continued)*	Amount	Cal.	Fat (g)	% Cal. Fat	Sat. Fat (g)	Trans Fat (g)	Chol. (mg)	Sod. (mg)	Carb. (g)	Fiber (g)	Pro. (g)	Choices/Exchanges
✔Cinnamon Dolce	12 oz	120	1	1	0	0	0	180	24	2	4	1 1/2 carb
Coffee	12 oz	180	3	2	1.5	0	10	170	37	0	4	2 1/2 carb
✔Espresso	12 oz	140	2	1	1	0	5	125	27	0	3	1 1/2 carb
✔Honey	12 oz	120	1	1	0	0	0	170	25	2	4	1 1/2 carb
✔Java Chip	12 oz	160	4	2	2	0	0	180	30	3	5	2 carb
Mint Mocha Chip	12 oz	170	3	2	1.5	0	0	180	32	3	5	2 carb
✔Mocha	12 oz	110	1	1	0	0	0	170	23	2	4	1 1/2 carb
✔Pumpkin Spice	12 oz	120	1	1	0	0	0	190	25	2	5	1 1/2 carb
✔White Chocolate Mocha	12 oz	140	2	1	1	0	0	190	27	2	5	2 carb
HOT ESPRESSO - 2% MILK												
Caffe Latte	12 oz	150	6	4	3.5	0	25	115	14	0	10	1 milk, 1 fat
Caffe Mocha - no whip	12 oz	200	6	3	3.5	0	20	100	31	1	10	1 carb, 1 milk, 1 fat

Item	Serving											Exchanges
Caffe Mocha - whip	12 oz	270	12	4	7	0	40	105	33	1	10	1 carb, 1 milk, 2 fat
✓Cappuccino	12 oz	90	4	4	2	0	15	70	9	0	6	1 milk, 1 fat
Peppermint White Chocolate Mocha - whip	12 oz	410	15	3	10	0	40	90	60	0	11	3 carb, 1 milk, 3 fat
✓Syrup Flavored Latte	12 oz	190	5	2	3.5	0	20	110	27	0	9	1 carb, 1 milk, 1 fat

HOT ESPRESSO - NONFAT

Item	Serving											Exchanges
✓Caffe Americano	12 oz	10	0	0	0	0	0	5	2	0	1	Free
✓Caffe Latte	12 oz	100	0	0	0	0	5	120	15	0	10	1 milk
✓Caffe Mocha - no whip	12 oz	170	2	1	0	0	5	100	32	1	10	1 carb, 1 milk
Caffe Mocha - whip	12 oz	230	8	3	4	0	25	110	34	1	11	1 carb, 1 milk, 1 1/2 fat
✓Cappuccino	12 oz	60	0	0	0	0	5	70	9	0	6	1 milk
✓Caramel Macchiato	12 oz	140	1	1	0.5	0	5	105	25	0	8	1 carb, 1 milk
Cinnamon Dolce Latte - no whip	12 oz	160	0	0	0	0	5	110	31	0	9	1 carb, 1 milk

✓ = Healthiest Bets

(Continued)

HOT ESPRESSO - NONFAT (Continued)

	Amount	Cal.	Fat (g)	% Cal. Fat	Sat. Fat (g)	Trans Fat (g)	Chol. (mg)	Sod. (mg)	Carb. (g)	Fiber (g)	Pro. (g)	Choices/Exchanges
✓ Cinnamon Dolce Latte - sugar free syrup	12 oz	90	0	0	0	0	5	125	14	0	9	1 milk
Cinnamon Dolce Latte - whip	12 oz	220	6	2	4	0	30	115	33	0	9	1 carb, 1 milk, 1 fat
Honey Latte - no whip	12 oz	160	0	0	0	0	5	115	31	0	9	1 carb, 1 milk
Honey Latte - whip	12 oz	220	6	2	4	0	30	120	33	0	9	1 carb, 1 milk, 1 fat
Peppermint White Chocolate Mocha - no whip	12 oz	320	5	1	3.5	0	5	180	59	0	11	3 carb, 1 milk
Peppermint White Chocolate Mocha - whip	12 oz	380	11	3	7	0	30	190	61	0	11	3 carb, 1 milk, 2 fat
Pumpkin Spice Latte - no whip	12 oz	200	0	0	0	0	5	170	38	0	11	1 1/2 carb, 1 milk
Pumpkin Spice Latte - whip	12 oz	260	6	2	4	0	30	170	40	0	11	1 1/2 carb, 1 milk, 1 fat

✔Skinny Caramel Latte - no whip	12 oz	90	0	0	0	5	125	14	0	9	1 milk
✔Skinny Cinnamon Dolce Latte - no whip	12 oz	90	0	0	0	5	125	14	0	9	1 milk
✔Skinny Hazelnut Latte - no whip	12 oz	90	0	0	0	5	125	14	0	9	1 milk
✔Skinny Mocha - no whip	12 oz	90	0	0	0	5	125	14	0	9	1 milk
✔Skinny Vanilla - no whip	12 oz	90	0	0	0	5	125	14	0	9	1 milk

HOT ESPRESSO - SOY

✔Caffe Latte	12 oz	130	4	3	0.5	0	100	18	1	7	1 milk, 1 fat
✔Caffe Mocha - no whip	12 oz	190	5	2	0.5	0	90	34	2	8	1 carb, 1 milk, 1 fat
Caffe Mocha - whip	12 oz	260	11	4	4.5	20	95	36	2	8	1 carb, 1 milk, 2 fat
✔Cappuccino	12 oz	80	3	3	0	0	60	11	1	4	1 milk, 1/2 fat
Peppermint White Chocolate Mocha - whip	12 oz	400	13	3	7	25	180	63	1	9	3 carb, 1 milk, 3 fat

✔ = Healthiest Bets

(Continued)

HOT ESPRESSO - SOY *(Continued)*	Amount	Cal. (g)	% Fat Fat	Sat. Cal. (g)	Trans Fat (g)	Fat (mg)	Chol. (mg)	Sod. (g)	Carb. (g)	Fiber (g)	Pro. Choices/Exchanges
Syrup Flavored Latte	12 oz	180	4	2	0.5	0	0	95	31	1	6	1 carb, 1 milk, 1 fat
HOT ESPRESSO - WHOLE MILK												
Caffe Latte	12 oz	180	9	5	5	0	30	115	14	0	10	1 milk, 2 fat
Caffe Mocha - no whip	12 oz	230	9	4	4.5	0	25	100	31	1	10	1 carb, 1 milk, 2 fat
Caffe Mocha - whip	12 oz	290	15	5	9	0	45	105	33	1	10	1 carb, 1 milk, 3 fat
Cappuccino	12 oz	110	6	5	3	0	15	70	9	0	6	1 milk, 1 fat
Peppermint White Chocolate Mocha - whip	12 oz	440	18	4	11	0	45	180	60	0	11	3 carb, 1 milk, 3 1/2 fat
Syrup Flavored Latte	12 oz	220	9	4	5	0	25	105	27	0	9	1 carb, 1 milk, 2 fat
ICED ESPRESSO - NONFAT												
✔Caffe Americano	12 oz	10	0	0	0	0	0	5	2	0	1	Free
✔Caffe Latte	12 oz	70	0	0	0	0	5	80	10	0	6	1 milk

✔ Caffe Mocha - no whip	12 oz	130	2	1	0	0	4	65	27	1	7	1 carb, 1 milk
Caffe Mocha - whip	12 oz	210	10	4	5	0	30	70	29	1	7	1 carb, 1 milk, 2 fat
✔ Caramel Macchiato - no whip	12 oz	140	1	1	1	0	5	100	25	0	7	1 carb, 1 milk
✔ Double shot + Energy Beverage	12 oz	70	0	0	0	0	0	15	14	0	3	1 carb
✔ Double shot Beverage	12 oz	60	0	0	0	0	0	15	14	0	2	1 carb
✔ Honey Latte - no whip	12 oz	130	0	0	0	0	5	70	25	0	6	1 carb, 1 milk
Honey Latte - whip	12 oz	210	8	3	5	0	35	80	28	0	6	1 carb, 1 milk, 1 1/2 fat
Peppermint White Chocolate Mocha - no whip	12 oz	280	5	2	3.5	0	5	140	54	0	7	3 carb, 1 milk
Peppermint White Chocolate Mocha - whip	12 oz	360	13	8	8	0	35	150	56	0	8	3 carb, 1 milk, 2 fat

(Continued)

✔ = Healthiest Bets

ICED ESPRESSO - NONFAT (Continued)	Amount	Cal.	Fat (g)	% Fat Fat	Sat. Fat Cal. (g)	Trans Fat (g)	Fat (mg)	Chol. (mg)	Sod. (g)	Carb. (g)	Fiber (g)	Pro. (g)	Choices/Exchanges
Pumpkin Spice Latte - no whip	12 oz	170	0	0	0	0	5	130	33	0	8	1 1/2 carb, 1 milk
Pumpkin Spice Latte - whip	12 oz	250	8	3	5	0	35	140	36	0	8	1 1/2 carb, 1 milk, 1 1/2 fat
✓Skinny Cinnamon Dolce Latte - no whip	12 oz	60	0	0	0	0	5	85	9	0	6	1 milk
✓Sugar-Free Syrup Flavored Latte	12 oz	60	0	0	0	0	5	85	9	0	6	1 milk
✓Syrup Flavored Latte	12 oz	120	0	0	0	0	0	90	24	0	6	1 carb, 1 milk
✓Vanilla Latte	12 oz	120	0	0	0	0	0	90	24	0	6	1 carb, 1 milk
White Chocolate Mocha - no whip	12 oz	230	5	2	3.5	0	5	150	42	0	8	2 carb, 1 milk
White Chocolate Mocha - whip	12 oz	320	12	3	8	0	35	160	44	0	9	2 carb, 1 milk, 2 fat

LOAVES AND COFFEE CAKES

Banana Nut Loaf	1 pc	470	23	4	3.5	0	40	220	59	3	5	4 carb, 4 1/2 fat
Classic Coffee Cake	1 pc	430	18	4	11	0	95	220	61	1	5	4 carb, 3 1/2 fat
Iced Lemon Pound Cake	1 pc	390	8	2	5	0	80	380	66	0	5	4 1/2 carb, 1 1/2 fat
No Sugar Added Banana Nut Coffee Cake	1 pc	480	28	5	4	0	45	210	63	3	7	4 carb, 5 1/2 fat
Pumpkin Loaf	1 pc	380	14	3	2	0	55	180	59	2	5	4 carb, 3 fat
Reduced Fat Banana Chocolate Chip Coffee Cake	1 pc	390	8	2	4.5	0	0	400	76	3	5	5 carb, 1 1/2 fat
Reduced Fat Blueberry Coffee Cake	1 pc	320	6	2	4.5	0	10	390	54	1	4	3 1/2 carb, 1 fat

MUFFINS AND SCONES

Blueberry Muffin	1	430	16	3	10	0	70	270	64	2	7	4 carb, 3 fat

✔ = Healthiest Bets

(Continued)

MUFFINS AND SCONES *(Continued)*	Amount	Cal.	Fat (g)	% Cal. Fat	Sat. Fat (g)	Trans Fat (g)	Chol. (mg)	Sod. (mg)	Carb. (g)	Fiber (g)	Pro. (g)	Choices/Exchanges
Blueberry Scone	1	500	23	4	13	0.5	75	640	68	2	7	4 1/2 carb, 4 1/2 fat
Bran Muffin	1	410	18	4	9	0	70	430	60	7	9	4 carb, 3 1/2 fat
Cranberry Orange Muffin	1	340	9	2	5	0	75	560	61	2	5	4 carb, 2 fat
Low Fat Blueberry Muffin	1	290	5	2	1	0	0	460	56	1	7	3 1/2 carb, 1 fat
Maple Oat Nut Scone	1	400	23	5	7	0	25	220	45	2	5	3 carb, 4 1/2 fat
✓Petite Vanilla Bean Scone	1	130	5	3	3	0	15	65	20	0	2	1 carb, 1 fat
Raspberry Scone	1	490	22	4	12	0.5	85	560	66	2	7	4 1/2 carb, 41/2 fat

TAZO TEA - NONFAT

	Amount	Cal.	Fat (g)	% Cal. Fat	Sat. Fat (g)	Trans Fat (g)	Chol. (mg)	Sod. (mg)	Carb. (g)	Fiber (g)	Pro. (g)	Choices/Exchanges
Iced Tazo Green Tea Latte	12 oz	160	0	0	0	0	5	85	32	1	7	2 carb
✓Tazo Black Shaken Iced Tea	12 oz	60	0	0	0	0	0	10	16	0	0	1 carb
✓Tazo Black Shaken Iced Tea Lemonade	12 oz	100	0	0	0	0	0	10	25	0	0	1 1/2 carb

Tazo Chai Iced Tea Latte	12 oz	150	0	0	0	5	70	33	0	5	2 carb
Tazo Chai Tea Latte	12 oz	150	0	0	0	5	75	33	0	6	2 carb
✓ Tazo Green Shaken Iced Tea	12 oz	60	0	0	0	0	10	16	0	0	1 carb
✓ Tazo Green Shaken Iced Tea Lemonade	12 oz	100	0	0	0	0	10	25	0	0	1 carb
✓ Tazo Green Tea Latte	12 oz	150	0	0	0	5	65	30	1	6	2 carb
✓ Tazo Passion Shaken Iced Tea	12 oz	60	0	0	0	0	10	16	0	0	1 carb
✓ Tazo Passion Shaken Iced Tea Lemonade	12 oz	100	0	0	0	0	10	25	0	0	1 1/2 carb
✓ Tazo Tea	12 oz	0	0	0	0	0	0	0	0	0	Free

✓ = Healthiest Bets

Subway
(www.subway.com)

Light 'n Lean Choice

Minestrone Soup *(8 oz)*
Ham Sandwich *(4")*
Oatmeal Raisin Cookie *(1)*

Calories	460	Cholesterol (mg)	25
Fat (g)	12	Sodium (mg)	2,005
% calories from fat	23	Carbohydrate (g)	75
Saturated fat (g)	5.5	Fiber (g)	9
Trans fat (g)	0	Protein (g)	18

Exchanges: 2 1/2 starch, 2 carb, 1 veg, 1 lean meat, 1 1/2 fat

Healthy 'n Hearty Choice

Chili Con Carne *(10 oz)*
Turkey Breast and Ham Sub *(6")*
Berry 'Lichus Fruizie Express *(small)*

Calories	690	Cholesterol (mg)	50
Fat (g)	13	Sodium (mg)	2,230
% calories from fat	17	Carbohydrate (g)	110
Saturated fat (g)	5	Fiber (g)	18
Trans fat (g)	0	Protein (g)	40

Exchanges: 5 1/2 starch, 2 carb, 1 veg, 2 1/2 medium-fat meat

Subway

	Amount	Cal.	Fat (g)	% Cal. Fat	Sat. Fat (g)	Trans Fat (g)	Chol. (mg)	Sod. (mg)	Carb. (g)	Fiber (g)	Pro. (g)	Choices/Exchanges
4″ SANDWICHES												
✔Ham	1	180	3	2	1	0	10	710	30	4	11	2 starch, 1 lean meat
✔Roast Beef	1	190	3.5	2	1.5	0	15	600	30	4	13	2 starch, 1 lean meat
✔Tuna w/Cheese	1	320	18	5	4.5	0	30	690	30	4	13	2 starch, 1 lean meat, 3 fat
✔Turkey Breast	1	190	3	1	1	0	15	670	30	4	12	2 starch, 1 lean meat
6″ DOUBLE SUBS (DOUBLE MEAT)												
Chicken & Bacon Ranch (includes cheese)	1	710	35	4	13	1	160	1890	48	6	55	3 starch, 6 medium-fat meat
Cold Cut Combo (includes cheese)	1	550	28	5	10	1	110	2360	49	5	31	3 1/2 starch, 3 medium-fat meat, 2 fat

✔ = Healthiest Bets

(Continued)

6" DOUBLE SUBS (DOUBLE MEAT) *(Continued)*	Amount	Cal.	Fat (g)	% Cal. Fat	Sat. Fat (g)	Trans Fat (g)	Chol. (mg)	Sod. (mg)	Carb. (g)	Fiber (g)	Pro. (g)	Choices/Exchanges
Ham	1	350	7	2	2.5	0	50	2020	49	5	28	3 1/2 starch, 2 lean meat
Italian BMT (includes cheese)	1	630	35	5	14	0	100	2850	49	5	34	3 1/2 starch, 3 medium-fat meat, 3 fat
Meatball Marinara (includes cheese)	1	860	42	4	18	2	85	2480	82	11	37	5 1/2 starch, 3 medium-fat meat, 5 fat
Oven Roasted Chicken Breast	1	400	8	2	2.5	0	45	1160	51	6	38	3 1/2 starch, 3 lean meat
Roast Beef	1	360	7	2	3.5	0	40	1300	46	5	29	3 starch, 3 lean meat
Steak & Cheese	1	540	18	3	8	1	105	1510	52	7	46	3 1/2 starch, 4 medium-fat meat
Subway Club	1	420	8	2	3.5	0	65	2080	50	5	39	3 1/2 starch, 3 lean meat
Subway Melt (includes cheese)	1	490	17	3	8	0	80	2500	51	5	40	3 1/2 starch, 3 medium-fat meat
Sweet Onion Chicken Teriyaki	1	480	7	1	2	0	100	1820	65	6	43	4 1/2 starch, 3 lean meat

Item	Amount	Cal.	Fat (g)	% Cal. Fat	Sat. Fat (g)	Trans Fat (g)	Chol. (mg)	Sodium (mg)	Carb. (g)	Fiber (g)	Pro. (g)	Exchanges/Choices
Turkey Breast	1	330	5		1	0	40	1500	48	5	28	3 starch, 2 lean meat
Turkey Breast & Ham	1	360	7		2	0	50	1930	50	5	31	3 1/2 starch, 2 lean meat

6" JARED SANDWICHES W/ 6G OF FAT OR LESS

Item	Amount	Cal.	Fat (g)	% Cal. Fat	Sat. Fat (g)	Trans Fat (g)	Chol. (mg)	Sodium (mg)	Carb. (g)	Fiber (g)	Pro. (g)	Exchanges/Choices
Ham	1	290	5	2	1.5	0	25	1260	47	5	18	3 starch, 1 lean meat, 1/2 fat
✓ Oven Roasted Chicken Breast	1	310	5	1	1.5	0	25	830	48	6	24	3 starch, 1 lean meat
✓ Roast Beef	1	290	5	2	2	0	20	900	45	5	19	3 starch, 1 lean meat
Subway Club	1	320	6	2	2	0	35	1290	47	5	24	3 starch, 2 lean meat
Sweet Onion Chicken Teriyaki	1	370	5	1	1.5	0	50	1200	59	5	26	4 starch, 1 lean meat
✓ Turkey Breast	1	280	5	2	1.5	0	20	1000	46	5	18	3 starch, 1 lean meat
✓ Turkey Breast & Ham	1	290	5	2	1.5	0	25	1210	47	5	20	3 starch, 1 lean meat
✓ Veggie Delite	1	230	3	1	1	0	0	500	44	5	9	3 starch, 1/2 fat

6" LIMITED TIME OFFER/REGIONAL SUBS

Item	Amount	Cal.	Fat (g)	% Cal. Fat	Sat. Fat (g)	Trans Fat (g)	Chol. (mg)	Sodium (mg)	Carb. (g)	Fiber (g)	Pro. (g)	Exchanges/Choices
Barbecue Chicken	1	310	6	2	2	0	35	1090	52	6	16	3 1/2 starch, 1 lean meat

(Continued)

✓ = Healthiest Bets

6" LIMITED TIME OFFER/ REGIONAL SUBS *(Continued)*	Amount	Cal.	Fat (g)	% Cal. Fat	Sat. Fat (g)	Trans Fat (g)	Chol. (mg)	Sod. (mg)	Carb. (g)	Fiber (g)	Pro. (g)	Choices/Exchanges
✔ Barbecue Rib Patty	1	420	19	4	6	0	50	810	47	5	20	3 starch, 2 medium-fat meat, 2 fat
Big Philly Cheese steak (double meat)	1	520	19	3	10	0	100	1390	50	6	40	3 1/2 starch, 4 medium-fat meat
✔ BLT (includes cheese)	1	350	13	3	6	0	30	940	43	5	18	3 starch, 1 medium-fat meat, 1 fat
Buffalo Chicken	1	380	18	4	4	0	55	1490	46	5	25	3 starch, 2 lean meat, 1 fat
The Feast (includes cheese)	1	590	25	4	10	0	105	3120	52	5	44	3 1/2 starch, 4 medium-fat meat
Pastrami (double meat)	1	580	30	5	10	0	14	1860	48	5	33	3 starch, 3 medium-fat meat, 2 fat
Subway Seafood Sensation (includes cheese)	1	450	22	4	6	1	25	1130	51	6	16	3 1/2 starch, 1 lean meat, 3 fat

6" SANDWICHES

Veggie Patty	1	390	8	2	1.5	0	10	1080	56	8	24	3 1/2 starch, 2 lean meat
Chicken & Bacon Ranch	1	580	30	5	11	1	99	1390	47	6	36	3 starch, 4 lean meat, 3 fat
Cold Cut Combo	1	410	17	4	7	0.5	60	1530	47	5	21	3 starch, 2 medium-fat meat, 1 fat
Italian BMT	1	450	21	4	8	0	55	1770	47	5	23	3 starch, 2 medium-fat meat, 2 fat
Meatball Marinara	1	560	24	4	11	1	45	1590	63	8	24	4 starch, 2 medium-fat meat, 3 fat
Spicy Italian	1	480	25	5	9	0	55	1660	45	5	21	3 starch, 2 medium-fat meat, 3 fat
Steak & Cheese	1	400	12	3	6	0.5	60	1110	48	6	29	3 starch, 2 medium-fat meat
Subway Melt	1	380	12	3	5	0	45	1600	48	5	25	3 starch, 2 medium-fat meat

✔ = Healthiest Bets

(Continued)

6" SANDWICHES *(Continued)*	Amount	Cal.	Fat (g)	% Cal. Fat	Sat. Fat (g)	Trans Fat (g)	Chol. (mg)	Sod. (mg)	Carb. (g)	Fiber (g)	Pro. (g)	Choices/Exchanges
Tuna	1	530	31	5	7	0.5	45	1010	44	5	22	3 starch, 2 lean meat, 5 fat
8" PIZZA												
Cheese	1	680	22	3	9	0	40	1070	96	4	32	6 1/2 starch, 1 medium-fat meat, 2 fat
Cheese & Veggies	1	740	25	3	11	0	50	1210	100	5	36	6 starch, 1 veg, 3 medium-fat meat, 2 fat
Pepperoni	1	790	32	4	13	0	60	1350	96	4	38	6 1/2 starch, 3 medium-fat meat, 3 fat
Sausage	1	820	34	4	14	0	68	1420	97	4	39	6 1/2 starch, 3 medium-fat meat, 3 fat
BREAKFAST SANDWICHES ON 6" BREAD												
Cheese	1	420	18	4	8	0	190	1010	44	5	23	3 starch, 2 medium-fat meat, 1 fat

Chipotle Steak & Cheese	1	600	32	5	11	0.5	220	1470	49	6	34
											3 1/2 starch, 3 medium-fat meat, 2 fat
Double Bacon & Cheese	1	510	25	4	11	0.5	210	1380	45	5	30
											3 starch, 3 medium-fat meat, 1 fat
Honey Mustard Ham & Cheese	1	470	19	4	8	0	200	1500	52	5	28
											3 1/2 starch, 3 lean meat, 2 fat
Western w/ Cheese	1	450	19	4	8	0	200	1390	46	5	28
											3 starch, 3 medium-fat meat, 1/2 fat

BREAKFAST WRAPS

Cheese	1	520	23	4	9	1	190	1260	55	2	25
											3 1/2 starch, 2 medium-fat meat, 2 fat
Chipotle Steak & Cheese	1	700	37	5	12	1	220	1720	60	3	35
											4 starch, 3 medium-fat meat, 3 fat
Double Bacon & Cheese	1	610	30	4	13	1	210	1630	56	2	30
											3 1/2 starch, 3 medium-fat meat, 3 fat

(Continued)

✔ = Healthiest Bets

BREAKFAST WRAPS *(Continued)*	Amount	Cal.	Fat (g)	% Cal. Fat	Sat. Fat (g)	Trans Fat (g)	Chol. (mg)	Sod. (mg)	Carb. (g)	Fiber (g)	Pro. (g)	Choices/Exchanges
Honey Mustard Ham & Cheese	1	580	25	4	10	1	200	1750	64	2	30	4 1/2 starch, 2 lean meat, 3 fat
Western w/ Cheese	1	550	24	4	10	1	200	1640	58	2	30	4 starch, 3 lean meat, 2 fat
CHEESE (AMOUNT ON 6" SUB, WRAP, OR SALAD)												
✔American, Processed	1 srvg	40	4	9	2	0	10	200	1	0	2	1 fat
✔Monterey Cheddar, Shredded	1 srvg	50	5	9	3	0	15	90	1	0	3	1 fat
✔Natural Cheddar	1 srvg	60	5	8	3	0	15	95	0	0	4	1 medium-fat meat, 1/2 fat
✔Pepperjack	1 srvg	50	4	7	2.5	0	15	140	0	0	3	1 fat
✔Provolone	1 srvg	50	4	7	2	0	10	125	0	0	4	1 medium-fat meat
✔Swiss	1 srvg	50	5	9	2.5	0	15	30	0	0	4	1 medium-fat meat, 1/2 fat

DESSERTS

Apple Pie	1 srvg	250	10	4	2	0	0	290	37	1	0	2 1/2 carb, 2 fat
✔Apple Slices	1 pkg	35	0	0	0	0	0	0	9	2	0	1/2 veg
✔Chocolate Chip Cookie	1	210	10	4	6	0	15	150	30	1	2	2 carb, 2 fat
✔Chocolate Chunk Cookie	1	220	10	4	5	0	10	100	30	<1	2	2 carb, 2 fat
✔Double Chocolate Chip Cookie	1	210	10	4	5	0	15	170	30	1	2	2 carb, 2 fat
M & M Cookie	1	210	10	4	5	0	10	100	32	<1	2	2 carb, 2 fat
✔Oatmeal Raisin Cookie	1	200	8	4	4	0	15	170	30	1	3	2 carb, 1 1/2 fat
Peanut Butter Cookie	1	220	12	5	5	0	15	200	26	1	4	1 1/2 carb, 2 1/2 fat
✔Raisins	1 pkg	140	0	0	0	0	0	0	33	2	2	2 veg
Sugar Cookie	1	220	12	5	6	0	15	140	28	<1	2	2 carb, 2 1/2 fat
White Chip Macadamia Nut Cookie	1	220	11	5	5	0	15	160	29	<1	2	2 carb, 2 fat

(Continued)

✔ = Healthiest Bets

DESSERTS *(Continued)*	Amount	Cal.	Fat (g)	% Cal. Fat	Sat. Fat (g)	Trans Fat (g)	Chol. (mg)	Sod. (mg)	Carb. (g)	Fiber (g)	Pro. (g)	Choices/Exchanges
✔Yogurt - Dannon All Natural Strawberry	4 oz.	110	1	1	0.5	0	5	65	20	0	5	1/2 carb, 1 milk

FRUIZLE EXPRESS

✔Berry Lishus	sm	110	0	0	0	0	0	30	28	1	1	2 carb
Berry Lishus w/Banana	sm	140	0	0	0	0	0	30	35	2	1	2 1/2 carb
✔Peach Pizzazz	sm	100	0	0	0	0	0	25	26	0	0	1 1/2 carb
Pineapple Delight	sm	130	0	0	0	0	0	25	33	1	1	2 carb
Pineapple Delight w/Banana	sm	160	0	0	0	0	0	25	40	2	1	2 1/2 carb
✔Sunrise Refresher	sm	120	0	0	0	0	0	20	29	1	1	2 carb

JARED LOW FAT FOOTLONG SANDWICHES

Ham	1	570	10	2	3.5	0	50	2520	93	11	37	6 starch, 2 lean meat
Oven Roasted Chicken Breast	1	630	11	2	3.5	0	45	1660	95	11	47	6 1/2 starch, 3 lean meat

	Amount	Cal	Fat (g)	% Cal. Fat	Sat. Fat (g)	Trans Fat (g)	Chol. (mg)	Sod. (mg)	Carb. (g)	Fiber (g)	Pro. (g)	Exchanges/Choices
Roast Beef	1	580	10	2	4.5	0	40	1800	90	11	38	6 starch, 2 lean meat, 1 fat
Subway Club	1	640	12	2	4.5	0	65	2580	94	11	48	6 1/2 starch, 3 lean meat
Sweet Onion Chicken Teriyaki	1	750	10	1	3	0	100	2400	118	11	52	8 starch, 3 lean meat
Turkey Breast	1	560	9	1	2.5	0	40	2000	92	11	37	6 starch, 2 lean meat
Turkey Breast & Ham	1	580	10	2	3	0	50	2420	93	11	40	6 starch, 2 lean meat
Veggie Delite	1	450	6	1	2	0	0	1000	88	11	18	6 starch, 1/2 fat
JARED SALADS W/ 6G OF FAT OR LESS												
✔ Ham	1	120	3	2	1	0	25	840	14	4	12	1 starch, 1 lean meat
✔ Oven Roasted Chicken Breast	1	140	3	2	0.5	0	50	390	11	4	19	1/2 starch, 1 lean meat
✔ Roast Beef	1	120	3	2	1.5	0	20	480	12	4	13	1 starch, 1 lean meat
✔ Subway Club	1	150	4	2	1.5	0	35	870	14	4	18	1 starch, 2 lean meat
✔ Sweet Onion Chicken Teriyaki	1	210	3	1	1	0	50	780	26	4	20	1 1/2 starch, 2 lean meat

(Continued)

✔ = Healthiest Bets

JARED SALADS W/ 6G OF FAT OR LESS *(Continued)*	Amount	Cal.	Fat (g)	% Cal. Fat	Sat. Fat (g)	Trans Fat (g)	Chol. (mg)	Sod. (mg)	Carb. (g)	Fiber (g)	Pro. (g)	Choices/Exchanges
✓Turkey Breast	1	110	3	2	0.5	0	20	580	13	4	12	1 starch, 1 lean meat
✓Turkey Breast & Ham	1	120	3	2	0.5	0	25	790	14	4	14	1 starch, 2 lean meat
✓Veggie Delite	1	60	1	2	0	0	0	80	11	4	3	1/2 starch
SALAD DRESSING												
Fat Free Italian	2 oz.	35	0	0	0	0	0	720	7	0	1	Free
Ranch	2 oz.	320	35	10	6	0.5	30	560	3	0	0	7 fat
SANDWICH CONDIMENTS (AMOUNT ON 6" SUB)												
Bacon	2 strips	45	4	8	1.5	0	10	190	0	0	3	1 fat
Chipotle Southwest Sauce	1 oz.	96	10	9	2	0	8	215	1	0	0	2 fat
Honey Mustard Sauce, Fat Free	1 oz.	30	0	0	0	0	0	115	7	0	0	1/2 carb
✓Light Mayonnaise	1 T	50	5	9	1	0	5	100	<1	0	0	1 fat

	Amount	Cal.	Fat (g)	% Cal. Fat	Sat. Fat (g)	Trans Fat (g)	Chol. (mg)	Sod. (mg)	Carb. (g)	Fiber (g)	Pro. (g)	Servings/Exchanges
Mayonnaise	1 T	110	12	10	2	0	10	80	0	0	0	2 1/2 fat
✔Mustard yellow or deli brown	2 tsp	5	0	0	0	0	0	115	<1	0	0	Free
Olive Oil Blend	1 tsp	45	5	10	0	0	0	0	0	0	0	1 fat
Ranch Dressing	1 oz.	120	13	10	2	0	10	210	1	0	0	2 1/2 fat
Red Wine Vinaigrette, Fat Free	1 oz.	29	0	0	0	0	1	340	6	0	0	Free
✔Sweet Onion Sauce, Fat Free	1 oz.	40	0	0	0	0	0	85	9	0	0	1/2 carb

SOUP

	Amount	Cal.	Fat (g)	% Cal. Fat	Sat. Fat (g)	Trans Fat (g)	Chol. (mg)	Sod. (mg)	Carb. (g)	Fiber (g)	Pro. (g)	Servings/Exchanges
Chicken and Dumpling	10 oz.	170	5	3	2	0	35	1390	23	2	8	1 1/2 starch, 1 fat
✔Chili con Carne	10 oz.	290	8	2	3.5	0	25	990	35	12	19	2 1/2 starch, 2 medium-fat meat
Cream of Broccoli	10 oz.	160	7	4	2.5	0	10	1010	18	5	6	1 starch, 1 1/2 fat

✔ = Healthiest Bets

(Continued)

SOUP *(Continued)*	Amount	Cal.	Fat (g)	% Cal. Fat	Sat. Fat (g)	Trans Fat (g)	Chol. (mg)	Sod. (mg)	Carb. (g)	Fiber (g)	Pro. (g)	Choices/Exchanges
Cream of Potato w/ Bacon	10 oz.	240	13	5	5	0	15	1050	26	3	5	1 1/2 starch, 2 1/2 fat
Golden Broccoli & Cheese	10 oz.	200	12	5	5	0	25	1180	17	3	5	1 starch, 2 1/2 fat
Minestrone	10 oz.	80	1	1	0.5	0	<5	1125	15	4	4	1 starch
✓New England Style Clam Chowder	10 oz.	150	5	3	1	0	10	990	20	4	6	1/2 starch, 1 milk, 1 fat
Roasted Chicken Noodle	10 oz.	80	2	2	0.5	0	15	1240	11	1	6	1/2 starch, 1 lean meat
Spanish Style Chicken w/ Rice	10 oz.	110	2	2	0.5	0	10	1300	17	1	6	1 starch, 1/2 fat
Tomato Garden Vegetable w/ Rotini	10 oz.	90	0	0	0	0	0	1140	20	2	3	1 starch, 1 veg
Vegetable Beef	10 oz.	100	2	2	0.5	0	10	1450	15	3	6	1 starch, 1/2 fat
Wild Rice w/ Chicken	10 oz.	210	11	5	4	0	25	1250	21	2	6	1 1/2 starch, 2 fat

VEGETABLES (AMOUNT ON 6" SUB)										
✔ Banana Peppers	3 rings		0	0	0	0	20	0	0	Free
✔ Cucumbers	3 slices	3	0	0	0	0	<1	0	0	Free
✔ Jalapeno Peppers	3 rings		3	0	0	0	70	0	0	Free
✔ Lettuce	1 srvg		3	0	0	0	0	0	0	Free
✔ Olives	3 rings		3	0	0	0	25	0	0	Free
✔ Onions	1 srvg	5	0	0	0	0	1	0	0	Free
✔ Pickles	3 chips		0	0	0	0	115	0	0	Free
✔ Tomatoes	3 wheels	5	0	0	0	0	2	0	0	Free

✔ = Healthiest Bets

Taco Bell
(www.tacobell.com)

Light 'n Lean Choice

Freso Menu: Beef Soft Taco (1)
Bean Burrito (1)
Salsa, side (1.5 oz, 3 Tbsp)

Calories	545	Cholesterol (mg)	25
Fat (g)	16	Sodium (mg)	2,000
% calories from fat	26	Carbohydrate (g)	78
Saturated fat (g)	6.5	Fiber (g)	11
Trans fat (g)	0.5	Protein (g)	21

Exchanges: 5 starch, 1/2 lean meat, 2 fat

Healthy 'n Hearty Choice

Gordita Supreme Steak (1)
Spicy Chicken Soft Taco (1)
Pintos 'n' Cheese (1 serving)

Calories	620	Cholesterol (mg)	80
Fat (g)	25	Sodium (mg)	1,780
% calories from fat	36	Carbohydrate (g)	67
Saturated fat (g)	10	Fiber (g)	11
Trans fat (g)	0.5	Protein (g)	34

Exchanges: 4 1/2 starch, 3 medium-fat meat, 2 fat

Taco Bell

BURRITOS

	Amount	Cal.	Fat (g)	Cal. Fat	Sat. Fat (g)	Trans Fat (g)	Chol. (mg)	Sod. (mg)	Carb. (g)	Fiber (g)	Pro. (g)	Choices/Exchanges
1/2 lb Beef & Potato Burrito	1	530	23	4	7	1	30	1720	66	6	15	4 1/2 starch, 4 fat
1/2 lb Beef Combo Burrito	1	440	18	4	7	1	45	1630	51	8	21	3 1/2 starch, 2 medium-fat meat, 1 1/2 fat
7-Layer Burrito	1	490	18	3	7	1	25	1350	65	9	17	4 1/2 starch, 1 medium-fat meat, 2 1/2 fat
Burrito Supreme - Beef	1	420	17	4	8	1	40	1340	51	7	17	3 1/2 starch, 1 medium-fat meat, 2 fat
Burrito Supreme - Chicken	1	400	13	3	6	0.5	45	1360	49	6	20	3 1/2 starch, 1 lean meat, 1 1/2 fat

(Continued)

✔ = Healthiest Bets

BURRITOS *(Continued)*	Amount	Cal.	Fat (g)	% Cal. Fat	Sat. Fat (g)	Trans Fat (g)	Chol. (mg)	Sod. (mg)	Carb. (g)	Fiber (g)	Pro. (g)	Choices/Exchanges
Burrito Supreme - Steak	1	390	14	3	6	1	40	1250	49	6	18	3 1/2 starch, 1 medium-fat meat, 1 fat
Fiesta Burrito - Beef	1	370	13	3	5	0	25	1200	49	4	14	3 1/2 starch, 1 medium-fat meat, 2 fat
Fiesta Burrito - Chicken	1	350	10	3	3.5	0	30	1220	47	3	18	3 starch, 1 lean meat, 1 fat
Fiesta Burrito - Steak	1	340	11	3	4	0	25	1110	47	3	15	3 starch, 1 medium-fat meat, 1 fat
Grilled Stuft Burrito - Beef	1	680	30	4	10	1	55	2120	76	9	27	5 starch, 2 medium-fat meat, 4 fat
Grilled Stuft Burrito - Chicken	1	640	23	3	7	0.5	65	2160	73	7	34	5 starch, 3 lean meat, 3 fat
Grilled Stuft Burrito - Steak	1	630	25	4	8	1	55	1930	72	7	30	5 starch, 2 medium-fat meat, 2 fat

Item	Amount	Cal.	Fat (g)	Sat. Fat (g)		Trans Fat (g)	Chol. (mg)	Sod. (mg)	Carb. (g)	Fiber (g)	Prot. (g)	Exchanges/Choices
Spicy Chicken Burrito	1	400	17	4	4	0	30	1190	48	3	14	3 starch, 1 lean meat, 3 fat

CHALUPAS

Item	Amount	Cal.	Fat (g)	Sat. Fat (g)		Trans Fat (g)	Chol. (mg)	Sod. (mg)	Carb. (g)	Fiber (g)	Prot. (g)	Exchanges/Choices
Chalupa Baja - Beef	1	410	27	6	6	0	35	780	30	4	13	2 starch, 1 medium-fat meat, 4 fat
Chalupa Baja - Chicken	1	390	23	5	4	0	40	800	29	3	17	2 starch, 2 lean meat, 3 1/2 fat
Chalupa Baja - Steak	1	390	24	6	4.5	0	35	690	28	3	15	2 starch, 1 medium-fat meat, 3 1/2 fat
Chalupa Nacho Cheese - Beef	1	370	22	5	4	0	20	770	32	3	12	2 starch, 1 medium-fat meat, 3 fat
✔Chalupa Nacho Cheese - Chicken	1	350	18	5	2	0	25	790	30	2	16	2 starch, 1 lean meat, 2 1/2 fat
✔Chalupa Nacho Cheese - Steak	1	340	19	5	2.5	0	20	670	30	2	14	2 starch, 1 medium-fat meat, 2 fat

(Continued)

✔ = Healthiest Bets

CHALUPAS *(Continued)*	Amount	Cal.	Fat (g)	% Cal. Fat	Sat. Fat (g)	Trans Fat (g)	Chol. (mg)	Sod. (mg)	Carb. (g)	Fiber (g)	Pro. (g)	Choices/Exchanges
✓Chalupa Supreme - Beef	1	380	23	5	7	0.5	40	620	30	3	14	2 starch, 1 medium-fat meat, 3 fat
✓Chalupa Supreme - Chicken	1	360	20	5	5	0	45	650	29	2	17	2 starch, 2 lean meat, 3 fat
Chalupa Supreme - Steak	1	360	21	5	6	0	40	530	28	2	15	2 starch, 1 medium-fat meat, 3 fat
FRESCO MENU												
Bean Burrito	1	330	7	2	2.5	0.5	0	1200	54	9	12	3 1/2 starch, 1 1/2 fat
Burrito Supreme - Chicken	1	330	8	2	2.5	0	25	1360	49	7	18	3 1/2 starch, 1 medium-fat meat, 1/2 fat
Burrito Supreme - Steak	1	330	8	2	3	0.5	20	1250	48	7	16	3 starch, 1 medium-fat meat, 1/2 fat
✓Crunchy Taco	1	150	8	5	2.5	0	20	370	13	3	7	1 starch, 1 medium-fat meat, 1 fat

Item	Amount	Cal.	Fat		Sat. Fat		Chol.	Sod.	Carb.		Prot.	Exchanges
Fiesta Burrito - Chicken	1	330	8	2	2.5	0	25	1240	48	3	16	3 starch, 1 lean meat, 1 fat
✔ Grilled Steak Soft Taco	1	160	5	3	1.5	0	20	550	20	2	10	1 1/2 starch, 1 medium-fat meat
✔ Ranchero Chicken Soft Taco	1	170	4	2	1.5	0	25	730	21	3	12	1 1/2 starch, 1 lean meat
✔ Soft Taco - Beef	1	180	7	4	3	0	20	650	21	3	8	1 1/2 starch, 1 medium-fat meat, 1 fat
Zesty Chicken Border Bowl w/o Dressing	1 srvg	350	8	2	1.5	0.5	25	1600	51	10	19	3 1/2 starch, 1 lean meat, 1 fat
GORDITAS												
Gordita Baja - Beef	1	340	19	5	5	0	35	780	29	4	13	2 starch, 1 medium-fat meat, 3 fat
Gordita Baja - Chicken	1	320	16	5	3.5	0	40	800	28	3	17	2 starch, 2 lean meat, 2 fat
Gordita Baja - Steak	1	320	17	5	4	0	35	690	27	3	15	2 starch, 1 medium-fat meat, 2 fat

(Continued)

✔ = Healthiest Bets

GORDITAS *(Continued)*	Amount	Cal.	Fat (g)	% Cal. Fat	Sat. Fat (g)	Trans Fat (g)	Chol. (mg)	Sod. (mg)	Carb. (g)	Fiber (g)	Pro. (g)	Choices/Exchanges
Gordita Nacho Cheese - Beef	1	300	14	4	3.5	0	20	770	31	3	12	2 starch, 1 medium-fat meat, 2 fat
✔Gordita Nacho Cheese - Chicken	1	280	11	4	2	0	25	790	29	2	16	2 starch, 1 lean meat, 1 1/2 fat
✔Gordita Nacho Cheese - Steak	1	270	12	4	2	0	20	680	29	2	14	2 starch, 1 medium-fat meat, 1 fat
Gordita Supreme - Beef	1	310	16	5	6	0.5	40	620	29	3	14	2 starch, 1 medium-fat meat, 2 fat
✔Gordita Supreme - Chicken	1	290	12	4	5	0	45	650	28	2	17	2 starch, 2 lean meat, 1 1/2 fat
Gordita Supreme - Steak	1	290	13	4	5	0	40	530	28	2	15	2 starch, 1 medium-fat meat, 1 1/2 fat

NACHOS

	Amount	Cal.	Fat (g)	% Cal. Fat	Sat. Fat (g)	Trans Fat (g)	Chol. (mg)	Sod. (mg)	Carb. (g)	Fiber (g)	Pro. (g)	Choices/Exchanges
Nachos	1 srvg	330	21	6	2	0	0	520	31	2	4	2 starch, 4 fat

	Serving	Cal.	Fat	Sat. Fat	Trans Fat	Chol.	Sod.	Carb.	Fiber	Pro.	Servings/Exchanges
Nachos BellGrande	1 srvg	770	44	5	8	1	30	1270	77	12	19	5 starch, 1 medium-fat meat, 8 fat
Nachos Supreme	1 srvg	440	26	5	6	1	30	790	40	7	12	2 1/2 starch, 1 medium-fat meat, 4 fat

REGIONAL MENU ITEMS

	Serving	Cal.	Fat	Sat. Fat	Trans Fat	Chol.	Sod.	Carb.	Fiber	Pro.	Servings/Exchanges
Cheese Quesadilla	1	470	26	5	12	0.5	50	1100	39	2	19	2 1/2 starch, 2 medium-fat meat, 3 1/2 fat
Chili Cheese Burrito	1	370	16	4	8	0.5	40	1060	40	3	16	2 1/2 starch, 1 medium-fat meat, 2 fat
✓Tostada	1 srvg	240	10	4	3.5	0.5	15	730	27	7	11	2 starch, 1 medium-fat meat, 1 fat

SIDES

	Serving	Cal.	Fat	Sat. Fat	Trans Fat	Chol.	Sod.	Carb.	Fiber	Pro.	Servings/Exchanges
Cheesy Fiesta Potatoes	1 srvg	290	17	5	3.5	0	15	830	29	2	4	2 starch, 3 1/2 fat
✓Mexican Rice	1 srvg	110	3	2	0	0	0	460	19	1	2	1 1/2 starch, 1/2 fat

(Continued)

✓ = Healthiest Bets

SIDES (Continued)	Amount	Cal.	Fat (g)	% Cal. Fat	Sat. Fat (g)	Trans Fat (g)	Chol. (mg)	Sod. (mg)	Carb. (g)	Fiber (g)	Pro. (g)	Choices/Exchanges
Pintos n Cheese	1 srvg	160	6	3	3	0.5	15	670	19	7	9	1 1/2 starch, 1 medium-fat meat, 1/2 fat
SPECIALTIES												
Chicken Fiesta Taco Salad	1 srvg	790	38	4	8	1	75	1830	77	13	37	4 starch, 3 veg, 4 lean meat, 5 fat
Chicken Fiesta Taco Salad w/o Shell	1 srvg	430	18	4	6	1	75	1560	38	11	30	1 starch, 3 veg, 4 lean meat, 1 1/2 fat
Chicken Quesadilla	1	520	28	5	12	0.5	75	1420	40	3	28	2 1/2 starch, 3 lean meat, 4 fat
Chicken Taquitos	1 srvg	310	11	3	4.5	0	40	980	37	2	18	2 1/2 starch, 2 lean meat, 1 1/2 fat
Crunchwrap Supreme	1	560	24	4	8	0.5	30	1430	68	5	17	4 1/2 starch, 4 1/2 fat
Enchirito - Beef	1	360	17	4	8	1	50	1420	34	7	18	2 1/2 starch, 2 medium-fat meat, 2 fat

Item	Amount											Servings/Exchanges
Enchirito - Chicken	1	340	13	3	7	0.5	50	1450	33	6	22	2 starch, 2 lean meat, 1 1/2 fat
Enchirito - Steak	1	330	14	4	7	1	45	1330	33	6	20	2 starch, 2 medium-fat meat, 1 fat
Express Taco Salad	1 srvg	610	32	5	10	1.5	65	1420	56	14	25	2 1/2 starch, 3 veg, 3 lean meat, 5 fat
Fiesta Taco Salad	1 srvg	840	45	5	11	1.5	65	1780	80	15	30	4 starch, 3 veg, 3 lean meat, 7 fat
Fiesta Taco Salad w/o Shell	1 srvg	470	24	5	10	1.5	65	1510	40	13	23	1 1/2 starch, 3 veg, 3 lean meat, 3 fat
✔Guacamole Side	1.5 oz.	70	5	6	1	0	0	180	5	2	1	1/2 starch, 1 fat
Mexican Pizza	1 srvg	530	30	5	8	1	40	1000	46	6	20	3 starch, 2 medium-fat meat, 4 fat
✔MexiMelt	1 srvg	280	14	5	7	0.5	40	860	22	3	15	1 1/2 starch, 2 medium-fat meat, 1 1/2 fat
✔Salsa Side	1.5 oz.	15	0	0	0	0	0	160	3	0	0	Free

(Continued)

✔ = Healthiest Bets

SPECIALTIES *(Continued)*	Amount	Cal.	Fat (g)	% Cal. Fat	Sat. Fat (g)	Trans Fat (g)	Chol. (mg)	Sod. (mg)	Carb. (g)	Fiber (g)	Pro. (g)	Choices/Exchanges
Sour Cream Side	1.5 oz.	80	7	8	4.5	0	25	30	3	0	1	1 1/2 fat
Southwest Steak Border Bowl	1 srvg	600	24	4	6	1	55	2120	68	9	28	4 1/2 starch, 2 medium-fat meat, 2 fat
Spicy Chicken Crunchwrap Supreme	1 wrap	540	23	4	7	0	40	1360	67	4	19	4 1/2 starch, 1 lean meat, 3 fat
Steak Quesadilla	1	520	28	5	13	1	70	1300	39	3	26	2 1/2 starch, 3 medium-fat meat, 3 fat
✔ Steak Taquitos	1 srvg	310	11	3	5	0	35	870	36	2	16	2 1/2 starch, 1 medium-fat meat, 1 fat
Zesty Chicken Border Bowl	1 srvg	640	35	5	6	1	30	1800	60	10	22	4 starch, 1 lean meat, 6 fat
Zesty Chicken Border Bowl w/o Dressing	1 srvg	440	15	3	2.5	0.5	30	1540	57	10	21	4 starch, 1 lean meat, 2 fat

TACOS

✔ Crunchy Taco Supreme	1	210	13	6	6	0.5	40	370	15	3	9	1 starch, 1 medium-fat meat, 1 1/2 fat
Double Decker Taco	1	320	13	4	5	0.5	25	810	38	6	14	2 1/2 starch, 1 medium-fat meat, 1 fat
Double Decker Taco Supreme	1	370	17	4	7	1	40	820	40	7	14	2 1/2 starch, 1 medium-fat meat, 2 fat
Grilled Steak Soft Taco	1	260	15	5	4.5	0	30	640	20	2	12	1 1/2 starch, 1 medium-fat meat, 2 fat
Ranchero Chicken Soft Taco	1	270	14	5	4	0	35	820	21	2	14	1 1/2 starch, 1 lean meat, 2 fat
Soft Taco Supreme - Beef	1	250	13	5	6	0.5	40	650	23	3	11	1 1/2 starch, 1 medium-fat meat, 1 1/2 fat
Spicy Chicken Soft Taco	1	170	6	3	2	0	25	580	20	2	10	1 1/2 starch, 1 lean meat, 1/2 fat

✔ = Healthiest Bets

(Continued)

VALUE MENU

	Amount	Cal.	Fat (g)	% Cal. Fat	Sat. Fat (g)	Trans Fat (g)	Chol. (mg)	Sod. (mg)	Carb. (g)	Fiber (g)	Pro. (g)	Choices/Exchanges
1/2 lb Cheesy Bean & Rice Burrito	1	470	20	4	5	0	10	1390	58	6	13	4 starch, 4 fat
Bean Burrito	1	350	9	2	3.5	0.5	5	1190	54	8	13	3 1/2 starch, 1 fat
Big Taste Taco	1	420	22	5	6	0	35	1030	43	4	14	3 starch, 1 medium-fat meat, 3 fat
Caramel Apple Empanada	1	290	15	5	2.5	0	0	270	38	2	3	2 1/2 carb, 2 fat
✓Cheese Roll-Up	1 srvg	200	10	5	5	0	20	490	19	1	9	1 1/2 starch, 1 medium-fat meat, 1 1/2 fat
Cheesy Double Beef Burrito	1	460	20	4	6	0.5	40	1610	52	5	18	3 1/2 starch, 1 medium-fat meat, 3 fat
✓Cinnamon Twists	1 srvg	170	7	4	0	0	0	200	26	1	1	1 1/2 carb, 1 fat

	Amount										Exchanges/Choices
✔Crunchy Taco	1	170	10	5	3.5	0	25	350	13	3	8	1 starch, 1 medium-fat meat, 1 fat
✔Soft Taco – Beef	1	200	9	4	4	0	25	630	21	3	10	1 1/2 starch, 1 medium-fat meat, 1 fat
Triple Layer Nachos	1 srvg	340	18	5	1.5	0	0	720	38	6	7	2 1/2 starch, 3 fat

✔ = Healthiest Bets

Wendy's
(www.wendys.com)

Light 'n Lean Choice

**Mandarin Chicken Salad with
Roasted Almonds *(1 packet)*
Low-Fat Honey Mustard *(1/2 packet, 2 Tbsp)*
Jr. Chocolate Frosty**

Calories	570	Cholesterol (mg)	100
Fat (g)	22	Sodium (mg)	1,055
% calories from fat	35	Carbohydrate (g)	59
Saturated fat (g)	5	Fiber (g)	5
Trans fat (g)	0	Protein (g)	34

Exchanges: 1/2 starch, 2 1/2 carb, 2 veg, 3 lean meat, 4 fat

Healthy 'n Hearty Choice

**Baked Potato, plain
Chili *(large)*
Side Salad with Light Classic
Ranch Dressing *(1 serving)***

Calories	675	Cholesterol (mg)	80
Fat (g)	35	Sodium (mg)	1,650
% calories from fat	47	Carbohydrate (g)	102
Saturated fat (g)	17	Fiber (g)	16
Trans fat (g)	5	Protein (g)	30

Exchanges: 6 starch, 1 veg, 2 medium-fat meat, 1 1/2 fat

Wendy's

	Amount	Cal.	Fat (g)	% Cal. Fat	Sat. Fat (g)	Trans Fat (g)	Chol. (mg)	Sod. (mg)	Carb. (g)	Fiber (g)	Pro. (g)	Choices/Exchanges
CHICKEN NUGGETS AND SAUCES												
✓Barbecue Sauce	1 order	45	0	0	0	0	0	160	11	0	1	1/2 carb
✓Chicken Nuggets	4 pcs	190	12	6	2	0	30	430	10	0	10	1/2 starch, 1 lean meat, 1 1/2 fat
✓Chicken Nuggets	5 pcs	230	15	6	3	0	35	420	12	0	12	1 starch, 1 lean meat, 2 fat
Chicken Nuggets	10 pcs	460	30	6	6	0	70	1040	24	0	24	1 1/2 starch, 3 lean meat, 4 1/2 fat
Heartland Ranch	1 order	160	17	10	2.5	0	15	220	1	0	0	3 1/2 fat
✓Honey Mustard	1 order	130	12	8	2	0	10	220	6	0	0	1/2 carb, 2 1/2 fat
✓Sweet & Sour	1 order	50	0	0	0	0	0	150	13	0	0	1 carb

✓ = Healthiest Bets

(Continued)

CHICKEN NUGGETS AND SAUCES *(Continued)*	Amount	Cal.	Fat (g)	% Cal. Fat	Sat. Fat (g)	Trans Fat (g)	Chol. (mg)	Sod. (mg)	Carb. (g)	Fiber (g)	Pro. (g)	Choices/Exchanges
FROSTY												
✓Chocolate	jr	160	4	2	2.5	0	15	75	26	0	4	1 1/2 carb, 1 fat
Chocolate	sm	320	8	2	5	0	35	150	52	0	9	3 1/2 carb, 1 1/2 fat
Chocolate	med	410	11	2	7	0.5	45	200	68	0	11	4 1/2 carb, 1 1/2 fat
Chocolate	lg	530	14	2	9	0.5	55	260	86	0	14	5 1/2 carb, 2 1/2 fat
Chocolate Fudge	sm	410	11	2	7	0.5	35	230	69	1	8	4 1/2 carb, 1 1/2 fat
Chocolate Fudge	lg	540	13	2	8	0.5	45	310	94	1	11	6 1/2 carb, 2 fat
Chocolate Twisted w/ M&M's	1	560	19	3	12	0.5	40	180	86	1	10	5 1/2 carb, 3 fat
Chocolate Twisted w/ Oreo	1	450	14	3	7	0	30	300	72	1	10	5 carb, 2 1/2 fat
Chocolate Twisted w/ Toll House Cookie Dough	1	480	16	3	10	0.5	35	220	77	1	10	5 carb, 2 1/2 fat

Strawberry	sm	390	11	3	7	0.5	35	170	67	0	7	4 1/2 carb, 1 1/2 fat
Strawberry	lg	520	13	4	8	0.5	45	220	91	0	9	6 carb, 2 fat
✔Vanilla	jr	150	4	2	2.5	0	20	90	26	0	4	1 1/2 carb, 1 fat
Vanilla	sm	310	8	2	5	0	35	180	52	0	8	3 1/2 carb, 1 1/2 fat
Vanilla	med	410	10	2	6	0.5	45	240	68	0	11	4 1/2 carb, 2 fat
Vanilla	lg	520	13	2	8	1	60	300	86	0	14	5 1/2 carb, 2 fat
Vanilla Bean	sm	380	11	3	7	0.5	35	170	65	0	7	4 1/2 carb, 1 1/2 fat
Vanilla Bean	lg	500	12	2	8	0.5	45	220	89	0	9	6 carb, 2 fat
Vanilla Float w/ Coca-Cola	1	380	7	2	4.5	0	30	160	75	0	7	5 carb, 1 fat
Vanilla Twisted w/ M&M's	1	550	19	3	12	0.5	40	210	86	1	10	5 1/2 carb, 3 fat
Vanilla Twisted w/ Oreo	1	440	14	3	6	0.5	35	320	72	1	9	5 carb, 2 1/2 fat
Vanilla Twisted w/ Toll House Cookie Dough	1	480	16	3	10	0.5	40	240	77	1	9	5 carb, 2 1/2 fat

(Continued)

✔ = Healthiest Bets

	Amount	Cal.	Fat (g)	% Cal. Fat	Sat. Fat (g)	Trans Fat (g)	Chol. (mg)	Sod. (mg)	Carb. (g)	Fiber (g)	Pro. (g)	Choices/Exchanges
SALAD DRESSINGS												
✔Balsamic Vinaigrette	1 srvg	90	6	6	1	0	0	380	8	0	0	1/2 carb, 1 fat
Chunky Blue Cheese	1 srvg	230	24	9	5	0	35	370	2	0	2	5 fat
Classic Ranch	1 srvg	200	20	9	3	0	15	340	3	0	1	4 fat
✔Fat Free French	1 srvg	70	0	0	0	0	0	170	17	1	0	1 carb
Italian Vinaigrette	1 srvg	130	11	8	1.5	0	0	320	8	0	6	1/2 carb, 2 fat
✔Light Classic Ranch	1 srvg	90	8	8	1.5	0	20	360	4	0	1	1/2 carb, 1 1/2 fat
Light Honey Dijon	1 srvg	100	5	5	1	0	20	280	13	1	1	1 carb, 1 fat
Thousand Island	1 srvg	290	28	9	4.5	0	30	530	9	0	1	1/2 carb, 5 1/2 fat
SALADS												
✔Caesar Salad	1	70	4	5	2	0	10	170	4	2	6	1 veg, 1 fat
✔Caesar Salad - Dressing	1 srvg	120	13	10	2	0	10	200	1	0	1	2 fat

Item	Amount	Cal	Fat (g)	% Cal. Fat	Sat. Fat (g)	Chol. (mg)	Sod. (mg)	Carb. (g)	Fiber (g)	Pro. (g)	Servings/Exchanges
Caesar Salad - Garlic Croutons	1 srvg	70	2.5	3	0	0	125	9	0	2	1/2 starch, 1/2 fat
Chicken BLT Salad	1	470	27	5	10	85	1280	23	3	35	1 starch, 3 veg, 5 lean meat, 2 fat
Chicken BLT Salad - Garlic Croutons	1 srvg	250	24	9	3.5	20	330	9	0	1	1/2 starch, 5 fat
✓ Chicken BLT Salad - Honey Dijon Dressing	1 srvg	70	3	4	0	0	125	9	0	2	1/2 carb, 1/2 fat
✓ Mandarin Chicken Salad	1	180	2	1	0.5	65	630	16	2	24	1/2 starch, 2 veg, 3 lean meat
✓ Mandarin Chicken Salad - Crispy Noodles	1 srvg	70	3	4	0	0	190	10	0	1	1/2 starch, 1 fat
✓ Mandarin Chicken Salad - Oriental Sesame Dressing	1 srvg	170	10	5	1.5	0	360	19	0	1	1 carb, 2 fat

(Continued)

✓ = Healthiest Bets

SALADS (Continued)	Amount	Cal.	Fat (g)	% Cal. Fat	Sat. Fat (g)	Trans Fat (g)	Chol. (mg)	Sod. (mg)	Carb. (g)	Fiber (g)	Pro. (g)	Choices/Exchanges
✔ Mandarin Chicken Salad - Roasted Almonds	1 srvg	130	11	8	1	0	0	70	4	2	5	2 fat
✔ Side Salad	1	35	0	0	0	0	0	25	8	2	1	1 veg
Southwest Taco Salad	1	400	22	5	12	1	85	1140	26	7	27	1 starch, 3 veg, 3 lean meat, 2 fat
✔ Southwest Taco Salad - Ancho Chipotle Dressing	1 srvg	90	8	8	2	0	10	240	3	0	1	1 1/2 fat
✔ Southwest Taco Salad - Sour Cream	1 srvg	45	4	8	2	0	10	25	2	0	1	1 fat
Southwest Taco Salad - Tortilla Strips	1 srvg	110	5	4	1	0	0	160	13	1	2	1 starch, 1 fat
SANDWICHES												
Baconator	1	840	51	5	23	2.5	195	1880	38	1	56	2 1/2 starch, 7 medium-fat meat, 3 1/2 fat

✓Cheeseburger, Kid's Meal	1	270	11	4	5	0.5	40	70	27	1	15	2 starch, 1 medium-fat meat, 1 fat
✓Crispy Chicken Sandwich	1	330	14	4	2.5	0	35	680	34	1	15	2 1/2 starch, 1 lean meat, 2 fat
Double w/ Everything and Cheese	1	710	40	5	17	2	160	1440	41	2	47	2 1/2 starch, 6 medium-fat meat, 2 1/2 fat
✓Grilled Chicken Go Wrap	1	260	11	4	3.5	0	45	760	23	1	17	1 1/2 starch, 2 lean meat, 1 fat
✓Hamburger, Kid's Meal	1	220	8	3	3	0	43	490	26	1	12	1 1/2 starch, 1 medium-fat meat, 1/2 fat
✓Homestyle Chicken Fillet Sandwich	1	430	16	5	2.5	0	45	1120	48	2	25	3 starch, 2 lean meat, 2 fat
✓Homestyle Chicken Go Wrap	1	320	15	4	4.5	0	35	860	29	1	15	2 starch, 1 lean meat, 2 fat
✓Jr. Bacon Cheeseburger	1	320	16	5	6	0.5	50	670	26	1	17	1 1/2 starch, 2 medium-fat meat, 1 1/2 fat

✓ = Healthiest Bets

(Continued)

292 *Wendy's*

SANDWICHES (Continued)	Amount	Cal.	Fat (g)	% Cal. Fat	Sat. Fat (g)	Trans Fat (g)	Chol. (mg)	Sod. (mg)	Carb. (g)	Fiber (g)	Pro. (g)	Choices/Exchanges
✔ Jr. Cheeseburger	1	270	11	4	5	0.5	10	360	27	1	15	2 starch, 1 medium-fat meat, 1 fat
✔ Jr. Cheeseburger Deluxe	1	300	14	4	6	0.5	45	730	29	2	15	2 starch, 1 medium-fat meat, 1 1/2 fat
✔ Jr. Hamburger	1	230	5	2	3	0	30	490	27	1	13	2 starch, 1 medium-fat meat
✔ Single w/ Everything	1	430	20	4	7	1	75	870	39	2	25	2 1/2 starch, 2 medium-fat meat, 1 1/2 fat
Spicy Chicken Filet Sandwich	1	440	16	3	2.5	0	60	1300	46	3	28	3 starch, 3 lean meat, 1 1/2 fat
✔ Spicy Chicken Go Wrap	1	320	16	5	4.5	0	43	960	28	2	17	2 starch, 2 lean meat, 2 fat
✔ Stack Attack	1	380	20	5	9	1	75	750	27	1	23	2 starch, 3 medium-fat meat, 1 1/2 fat

Triple w/ Everything and Cheese	1	980	60	6	27	3.5	245	2010	43	2	69	3 starch, 9 medium-fat meat, 3 1/2 fat
✔Ultimate Chicken Grill Sandwich	1	320	7	2	1.5	0	70	952	36	2	28	2 1/2 starch, 3 lean meat

SIDE SELECTIONS

✔Baked Potato - Plain	1	270	0	0	0	0	0	25	61	7	7	4 starch
✔Baked Potato - Sour Cream & Chive	1	320	4	1	2	0	10	50	63	7	8	4 starch, 1 fat
Chili	sm	190	6	3	2.5	0	40	830	19	5	14	1 1/2 starch, 1 medium-fat meat
Chili	lg	280	9	3	3.5	0.5	60	1240	29	7	21	2 starch, 2 medium-fat meat
✔Chili - Saltine Crackers	1 order	25	1	4	0	0	0	95	4	0	0	Free
✔Chili - Seasoning	1 order	5	0	0	0	0	0	270	1	0	0	Free

✔ = Healthiest Bets

(Continued)

SIDE SELECTIONS *(Continued)*	Amount	Cal.	Fat (g)	% Cal. Fat	Sat. Fat (g)	Trans Fat (g)	Chol. (mg)	Sod. (mg)	Carb. (g)	Fiber (g)	Pro. (g)	Choices/Exchanges
Chili - Shredded Cheddar Cheese	1 order	70	6	8	3.5	0	15	110	1	0	4	1 fat
✔French Fries	kid's	210	10	4	1.5	0	0	180	28	3	3	2 starch, 2 fat
French Fries	small	340	16	4	2.5	0	0	290	45	4	4	3 starch, 3 fat
French Fries	med	430	20	4	3	0	0	370	56	5	6	4 starch, 3 1/2 fat
French Fries	lg	550	26	4	4	0	0	480	72	7	7	5 starch, 4 fat
✔Mandarin Orange Cup	1	80	0	0	0	0	0	15	19	1	1	1 fruit

✔ = Healthiest Bets